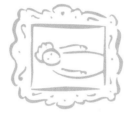

The Pregnancy Journal

A Day-to-Day Guide to a
Healthy and Happy Pregnancy

A. CHRISTINE HARRIS, PH.D.

ILLUSTRATIONS BY GREG STADLER

CHRONICLE BOOKS
SAN FRANCISCO

To my own precious family: my husband, Bob; daughter Heather;

her husband, Ryan Carroll; and our grandchildren, Olivia (9) and Colt (7).

In 2011 we became parents again by adopting granddaughters

Alexis Madiscella Ayala (19) and Isabella Ariceli Bautista-Harris (12).

We are so lucky to have such a great family!

This Chronicle Books LLC edition published in 2016.
Text copyright © 1996, 2009, 2016 by A. Christine Harris.
Illustrations copyright © 1996, 2009, 2016 by Greg Stadler.

Library of Congress Cataloging-in-Publication Data

Names: Harris, A. Christine.
Title: The pregnancy journal : a day-to-day guide to a healthy and happy
   pregnancy / A. Christine Harris, Ph.D. ; illustrations by Greg Stadler.
Description: Chronicle Books LLC edition, 4th edition. | San Francisco, CA :
   Chronicle Books LLC, 2016. | Includes index.
Identifiers: LCCN 2015050260 | ISBN 9781452155524 (pbk. : alk. paper)
Subjects: LCSH: Pregnancy—Popular works. | Pregnancy—Miscellanea.
Classification: LCC RG525 .H357 2016 | DDC 618.2—dc23 LC record available at http://lccn.loc
.gov/2015050260

Manufactured in China

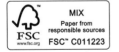

Design by Gretchen Scoble
Illustrations by Greg Stadler

10 9 8 7 6 5 4 3 2 1

Chronicle Books LLC
680 Second Street
San Francisco, CA 94107
www.chroniclebooks.com

CONTENTS

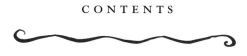

PREFACE

When I was pregnant with my two daughters Heather (the elder by three years) and Wendy, I was amazed by the transformative properties of pregnancy. I felt different, in many ways physically better than usual and "special" because I was carrying a child. But there were also some surprises: I felt unusually tired, even with normal rest, and I worried more than I thought I would. I was also surprised that I could apply so little of my knowledge about prenatal development and human behavior to my own pregnancy.

My practitioners offered good care, but their answers to my questions about my baby's development always seemed vague: "How's my baby doing?" I would ask. "Fine," they would say. "I can hear the baby's heartbeat." I longed to know more: What features were present? Could my baby move around? Was my baby processing any sensory information? How much did the baby weigh? Where was my baby in terms of development?

I eventually found the answers to these questions while doing research for a textbook on child development. Those answers, too late to provide insight into the chronology of my own pregnancies, are summarized within the pages of this book. Thus, it is my hope that *The Pregnancy Journal* will help parents feel:

- **enlightened and inspired about their baby and their pregnancy**
- **informed about how pregnancy can influence their bodies, themselves, and those around them**
- **a sense of wonder and amazement as they follow the fascinating chronology of their baby's cell-by-cell growth**
- **inspired to act in the best interests of their baby during and after pregnancy**
- **a powerful emotional connection to their son(s) and/or daughter(s) that manifests as deep and abiding affection, fascination, and sheer delight**
- **inspired to make a lifetime commitment to prioritizing their baby's needs above their own**

The Pregnancy Journal is keyed to your baby's birthday (due date), so your son's or daughter's personal day-by-day growth is laid out like a daily planner. No need to sit down and digest an entire chapter before you guess how it might apply to your own baby at any particular time. The developmental entries are brief enough to be read quickly and easily with key information in **bold print.** In addition, the recommendations and revelations are thorough, current, interesting, and derived from evidence-based knowledge and best practices.

The space set aside for recording your thoughts, hopes, and special memories of this pregnancy and the amazing baby that you will soon meet and raise make this journal even more individualized. There is room to record what you want to be sure to remember about a particular day, week, or month. There are sections called "Time to Reflect," where a writing prompt might ask: When did you begin to think about having this baby? What are you especially excited about right now?

or What's one thing that you do for your baby every day without fail? And there are places to list and compare progressive changes in your waist size and weight. One day you can share your responses and special memories with your child to complete his or her understanding of their life before birth. And what a unique opportunity for you to relive the feelings and experiences that created the story of your child's birth!

Extensive content revisions have been incorporated into this twentieth anniversary edition. Reliable research findings add new knowledge and validate or refine past practices. In order to give your baby every developmental advantage, you can rest assured that all recommendations are up-to-date and current.

Many women read *The Pregnancy Journal* with their husband, wife, partner, special friend, or their own mother, father, or parent figure. I would encourage you to do the same. Enjoy! Share! Communicate! Each pregnancy is a once-in-a-lifetime experience for all participants. In retrospect, the time between conception and birth comes and goes in the blink of an eye.

A. Christine Harris, Ph.D.

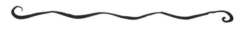

ACKNOWLEDGMENTS

I am grateful for the support, encouragement, and good advice of a fine collection of people. First and foremost, my family is utterly patient and supportive. In am indebted to my husband, Bob Harris, for doing everything a great partner needs to do to encourage my progress, shore up my energy, and offer advice. When I need a lift, sister Debby Day Carman, "Nana" Jeanne Carroll, daughter Heather, sister Care, my four grandchildren, sister Diana, son-in-law Ryan, and my flowers never let me down.

When she was in the sixth grade, my daughter Heather Harris (Carroll) thought the book sounded like a great idea and her validation really got the project off the ground. Next, my talented sister Carolyn Johnson used her creativity and graphic arts skills to transform the lifeless text into an eye-catching document. Finally, and through an incredible stroke of luck, colleague Cath Hooper, pregnant with her first child Theo, became intrigued and helped me establish a rewarding working relationship with Chronicle Books through Rob Shaeffer, Karen Silver, and Ursula Cary. *The Pregnancy Journal* and Chronicle Books have now been partnered for more than twenty years. Most recently, I have enjoyed working with Chronicle's Christine Carswell, Lorena Jones, Laura Lee Mattingly, and Leigh Saffold.

Finally, great friends and colleagues continue to be important to me and my work. I'm particularly grateful for Clyde Perlee Jr., John Davis, Bill Karns, Karen Andrew, Cathy Kennedy, Becky Pellegrin, Barbara Mitchell, Socorro Molina, Claire O'Connor, Mattie Cook, Phyllis Ramsey, Mrs. Jessie Andrews, and Lynn Fowler.

Personalizing The Pregnancy Journal

All of the information in this journal is keyed to your estimated due date, or EDD. In that way, the information is not just a description of the sequence of events for any pregnancy; it's the sequence of events for your unique pregnancy.

The easiest way to personalize *The Pregnancy Journal* is to begin with your baby's current due date, Journal Day 266. First, open the book to Day 266 (page 179) and write your baby's due date on that day. Then, using a monthly calendar as a guide and working backward from Journal Day 266, date each day in reverse sequence.

For example, if your baby's due date is January 2:

Day 266 = January 2

Day 265 = January 1

Day 264 = December 31

Mark the days all the way back to Journal Day 1, the approximate day your baby was conceived.

Women who undergo in vitro fertilization or artificial insemination know the actual date of conception. If this is the case, write the date of your baby's conception on Journal Day 1 and work forward. Date each day using a monthly calendar as a guide.

For simplicity's sake, the medical profession actually counts the 2 weeks that set the stage for conception as part of "the pregnancy" by asking you to remember back to the first day of your last normal menstrual period (LMP). Thus, your doctor's estimate seems ahead by 2 weeks because of its earlier starting point. Going back 38 weeks from the baby's due date (266 days) takes you back to the estimated day of conception; going back 40 weeks from the baby's due date (280 days) takes you back to the first day of your last menstrual cycle. In both cases, the due date remains the same. For your convenience, the LMP time frame your practitioner typically uses is also included.

Now that you have personalized your journal, you will be able to follow the unfolding events of your baby's development and your pregnancy by using the journal like a daily planner. You can read about your baby's growth for today's date, look ahead to see what you can expect, and look back to see what has already taken place.

Lunar Month 1

Development is measured in lunar months, not calendar months, to correspond to the menstrual cycle. Each lunar month consists of 28 days organized into four weeks of 7 days each.

THINGS TO DO THIS MONTH:

* Eat foods from clean, healthy sources, preferably fresh foods that are organically grown.

* Make sure you are getting plenty of protein, calcium, folic acid, zinc, vitamin A, B-complex vitamins, trace elements, phytonutrients, and bioflavonoids.

* Concentrate on incorporating superfoods into your diet: broccoli, kale, kidney beans, black beans, green tea, spinach, tomatoes, walnuts, sweet potatoes, wild salmon, and oats.

* Eat complex carbohydrates.

* Avoid processed and fast food.

* Eat foods with omega-3 fatty acids and omega-6 fatty acids regularly.

* Avoid foods containing trans fats, and limit saturated fats, to raise your HDL levels.

* Check the safety of herbal beverages and dietary supplements.

* Limit/avoid caffeine.

* Walk daily.

* Get sufficient rest.

* **Absolutely no smoking, alcohol, or drugs.**

* Check over-the-counter medicines with your health-care provider before you use them.

* Combat nausea associated with low blood sugar by eating small meals every two hours and having a snack at bedtime and waking.

* Combat nausea associated with odor sensitivity with natural peppermint, spearmint, lemon balm tea, and vitamin B_6 (check the dosage with your practitioner). Also avoid odors that bother you.

* Drink 13 cups (3 liters) of fluids per day between meals; always have water with you.

* Avoid viral illness.

* Contact your health-care provider if you experience vaginal bleeding, pelvic or lower abdominal pain, or persistent backache.

The Beginning

DAY 1	DATE:
	265 days to go

Today, a single-cell organism forms from the union of your egg (ovum) and your partner's sperm. Over the coming months, your daughter or son will develop from this barely **visible single cell** called a zygote. This beginning is called **conception or fertilization.**

As you think back, do you remember this date? Some women can feel when they ovulate, others can't. (It's okay either way.) It actually takes the sperm about 12 hours to reach the egg, which is in the uterine tube (the tube that connects the ovaries with the uterus) when the sperm begin to arrive. Although hundreds of sperm may swarm the egg, only one will penetrate the egg's outer surface. While this process of fertilization involves a tremendous amount of activity by the involved cells, **you are as unaware of the event of fertilization as you are the routine production of red blood cells by your system.**

For Your Information The lengthy travel time required by the sperm is what establishes the **time that women can usually get pregnant** at five days before ovulation and the day of ovulation.

Did You Know? Each zygote is genetically unique, even in the case of identical twins.

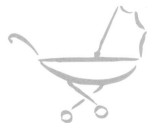

DAY 2	DATE:
	264 days to go

The **first cell division** takes place today. A two-cell ball is formed from the single cell created by your ovum and your partner's sperm. This cell ball floats freely in the uterine tube, pushed along by gravity and the movement of the tiny hairs (cilia) that line that tube.

Early Pregnancy Factor (EPF), a protein that fights off your body's natural defenses against cells that are unlike your own, is first manufactured now. Without EPF, your body might mistake the developing baby for a foreign body like a virus and attack it. With EPF, your baby can continue to develop without risk.

IMPORTANT: Of all the factors that affect pregnancy outcomes, nutrition is the most important and the easiest to modify. A nutritious diet of the purest and most natural foods directly benefits your health and your baby's development and future health, and contributes to a healthy ecosystem. **The most critical nutrients** are protein, calcium, folic acid, iron, zinc, vitamin A, the B-complex vitamins, vitamin C, and the trace elements, phytonutrients, and bioflavonoids contained in natural foods.

Chart your **waist size and weight** here and on page 181. This first measurement is very important. You'll have fun looking back and comparing each of the measurements with the ones that preceded.

WAIST SIZE   WEIGHT
....

Nothing is worth more than this day.

J. W. GOETHE

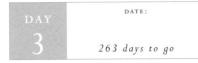

DAY 3	DATE:
	263 days to go

In the last 24 hours, two identical cells have undergone three or four additional cell divisions. Two cells become four, four cells become eight, and eight cells become sixteen and take the shape of a tightly packed, solid ball. Because the original cell is dividing into smaller units, there is little or no increase in your baby's total size.

The baby's cells are manufactured now by relying on the **nutrients found in the "yolk sac" of your egg.**

Food Facts **Folic acid or vitamin B$_9$ is a critically important nutrient** for women in their childbearing years—ages 12–13 (first menstrual period) to age 50 (average age of menopause). During pregnancy, it's involved in every body function that involves cell division, creates the DNA molecule, and helps safeguard the development of the brain and nervous system. Folic acid also works with vitamins B$_{12}$ and C to help your baby's body digest, use, and produce proteins. The recommended daily dose of folic acid during pregnancy is 600 mcg. The folate supplements and fortified foods are actually absorbed better than the natural form in foods.

What do you want to be sure to remember?

_____

_____

_____

_____

(See page 28 for more space to write.)

DAY 4	DATE:
	262 days to go

The 16-cell solid ball has reached the end of your uterine tube. **It will soon get some nourishment from the tissue that lines the uterus (endometrium), which releases high levels of fats and sugars.** In turn, the cell ball itself releases a very sticky substance. This coating helps it hold fast to the surface of the uterus so it can push itself deep inside.

The ball of cells that was once the fertilized egg is making slow progress. **It will enter your uterus either today or tomorrow.**

For Your Information **Protein provides amino acids, which are required to build everything in your baby's body**—from brain chemicals to muscles to antibodies. Most pregnant women in the United States don't need to add protein-rich foods to their diet to consume the recommended 71 g of protein per day. But they do need to consume protein from cleaner, sustainable sources. For example, organic poultry without the skin (turkey is the leanest); fortified eggs; hormone-free lean meat; clean, sustainable sources of fish and shellfish; soy—especially tofu, tempeh, soy milk, and edamame; nuts; dried beans and peas; and grains—all produced by organic agriculture that aims to reduce the use of toxic chemicals—are high-quality protein sources.

There is no finer investment for any community than putting milk into babies.
WINSTON CHURCHILL

DAY 5	DATE:
	261 days to go

An important change takes place in the cell ball. Fluid secreted by the cells passes into the center of the cell ball and divides the cells into two groups: Those on the outside will support the pregnancy, and those on the inside will form the baby.

If the cell ball hasn't already entered your uterus, it will do so today. **Your body still doesn't realize your baby exists**, since EPF is secreted by the cell ball.

Did You Know? **Women need twice as much iron—27 mg per day—during pregnancy.** The amount of blood the pregnant woman's body produces increases by 50 percent and every red blood cell uses iron, as does the baby and the placenta. In addition, about one-third of women's stored iron will be passed to her baby to make its own red blood cells and to start its own reserve for future use. Most women don't start pregnancy with sufficient amounts of stored iron. Therefore, many women take an iron supplement, since they can't reliably bring their iron levels up through diet alone.

DAY 6	DATE:
	260 days to go

If fluid hasn't already passed into the center of the cell ball to divide it into two groups of cells, it will do so today. The fluid-filled cell ball rests on the sticky surface of your uterus. **The cell ball now contains several hundred cells**, some of which group together to form a bump on the inside of the ball.

When the cell ball comes to rest on the surface of your uterus, the process of implantation begins. During implantation, the outer cells that have made contact literally fuse with the cells on the surface of your uterus. **Implantation establishes the pregnancy** by providing your baby-ball with oxygen and nutrients from your bloodstream.

Did You Know? Some of the **early signs of pregnancy** include tingling or tenderness of the breasts or nipples, nausea, extreme fatigue, and lack of a period or frequent spotting. Breast changes may be difficult to detect if you're still nursing from a previous pregnancy or have just finished.

Food Facts **Processing takes nutrients away from foods.** Fresh foods have higher nutritional value than frozen or canned foods. Eat local, seasonal, fresh foods. Roasting, steaming, or microwaving helps retain the foods' vitamins, minerals, and antioxidant compounds. Add fresh, natural veggies to soups, pasta, rice, stews, stir-fries, and egg dishes.

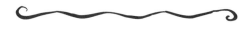

TIME TO REFLECT
Was your pregnancy planned or a surprise?

_____

_____

_____

_____

_____

_____

_____

_____

It goes without saying that you should never have more children than you have car windows.
ERMA BOMBECK

| DAY 7 | DATE:

259 days to go |

Implantation continues. The actual size of the implanted cell ball is 0.004 inch (0.1 mm). Ten implanted cell balls could fit into the space occupying the period at the end of this sentence. **What's more, your baby is one week old already!**

When implantation is taking place, the cell ball actually burrows into your uterine lining. As a result, you may notice some menstrual-like cramping and spotting. **(Don't mistake this for a light period.)** Because of hormonal changes, some of the other early signs of pregnancy include tingling or tenderness of the breasts or nipples, extreme fatigue, and nausea.

IMPORTANT: Before you drink products labeled **"Pregnancy Tea,"** check the ingredients list with your health care provider. Raspberry leaf tea may be safe to drink after Week 30/LMP Week 32 since it can stimulate and strengthen your uterus. Decaffeinated versions of non-herbal teas (black, green, and oolong) still contain a bit of caffeine.

Food Facts **Superfoods** are considered so nutritionally well rounded and packed with phytonutrients that they should be part of every healthy diet. While there is no official definition of a superfood, broccoli, kale, spinach, wild salmon, and walnuts seem to be on everyone's list. Other top-drawer foods: beans (especially black and kidney), decaffeinated green tea, sweet potatoes, tomatoes, and oats.

Did You Know? Building a baby is like building a house—the framework precedes the details, and the foundation sets the tone for the lifetime of the structure. **Now is the time to do everything in your power to have a healthy baby.**

What do you want to be sure to remember?

(See page 28 for more space to write.)

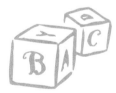

I'll love you forever, I'll like you for always. As long as I'm living, my baby you'll be.
ROBERT MUNSCH

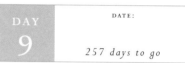

LMP Week 4

DAY 8	DATE:
	258 days to go

The surface of the cell ball secretes a substance that breaks down uterine tissue to form a little "cave" for itself under the surface. Once nestled into its cave, the cell ball anchors itself to the uterus by creating **root-like structures called villi.** Once implantation is complete, the developing baby is called an *embryo*, from the Greek words meaning "to grow in" (*en* = in and *bruein* = to grow).

Congratulations! You (actually, your body) have finally officially met your developing baby. The two of you are now intimately joined, and **your body begins to mobilize to support your baby's growth.** You don't realize it yet, but you've been pregnant for a whole week!

Did You Know? **The embryonic baby is a self-contained unit that plays a role in creating its own environment.** For example, its delicate tissues must be constantly bathed in fluids or they would dry out or be crushed. Your body anticipates this need. Even before the embryo is formed, some cells gather to make a transparent bubble. Fluid seeps into the bubble from surrounding maternal tissues and the bubble becomes the amniotic sac containing amniotic fluid. (The word *amnion* is from a Greek word meaning "little lamb"; lambs are often born surrounded by their prenatal "bubble," or amniotic sac.)

DAY 9	DATE:
	257 days to go

By now the embryo has actually sunk beneath the surface of your uterus. The *amniotic sac* (the water-tight bag of waters) and the *amniotic cavity* (the area within the womb that contains the amniotic sac, amniotic fluid, and the developing child) begin to form. The amniotic sac and amniotic cavity require the next six days to complete their initial formation. The yolk sac has been emptied of its nutrients like emptying a bathtub. **A primitive version of the umbilical cord, called the umbilical stalk, appears.**

The placenta usually forms at the bottom of the implantation cave from tissue contributed by both you and your baby. Many spiral arteries from the lining of your uterus penetrate the placenta from the maternal side and open into the spaces between the "roots." **The main exchange of blood between you and your baby takes place through the walls of these little roots.**

For Your Information **The yolk sac fills up again, this time with fluid, and eventually gives rise to the baby's digestive tract.** (Wow! Your baby is just nine days old and recycling already!)

Did You Know? Prenatal growth is an amazing process. Your baby's mouth, spinal cord, and anus are the first structures formed. Once they are placed in a straight line, development proceeds around them.

A baby is God's opinion that life should go on.
CARL SANDBURG

<table>
<tr><td>DAY
10</td><td>DATE:

256 days to go</td></tr>
</table>

 Implantation is now complete and the placenta begins to function. Your embryonic baby grows rapidly. The amniotic sac, amniotic cavity, umbilical cord, and yolk sac continue to develop.

Good personal health habits have never been as important as they are now. If you are the type of person who already eats healthy, well-balanced meals, exercises moderately, gets sufficient rest, and does not smoke, drink alcohol, or take drugs, stay the course. Any positive change at any time during the pregnancy—especially early on—**directly benefits your baby for the rest of his or her life.**

Food Facts **Vitamin B$_{12}$ is a critical nutrient.** It helps folic acid manufacture new cells and is also needed to make DNA, the genetic material in each cell. B$_{12}$ also protects nerve fibers, promotes nervous system growth, and helps produce red blood cells. A daily intake of 2.6 mcg of vitamin B$_{12}$ is recommended during pregnancy. Anyone who makes healthy food choices regarding hormone-free meat, poultry, fortified eggs, natural cheese or organic milk products on a daily basis is guaranteed an adequate intake. Strict vegetarians can supplement their diets or drink vitamin B$_{12}$–fortified soy milk.

Did You Know? With the exception of B$_{12}$, most vitamins are stored in the body only in small amounts. **Vitamin B$_{12}$ is crucial to brain and major organ formation and function.** So much so that the body builds up stores that can last several years after the intake of the vitamin stops.

For Your Information Cells at the implantation site secrete *hCG*, a hormone that plays an important role in pregnancy. Currently, the most sensitive home pregnancy tests can detect the presence of hCG by today, Day 10. A negative result does not rule out the possibility of pregnancy when testing this early, so be sure to retest on the first day of your missed menstrual period. **Follow-up testing by your practitioner is a must!**

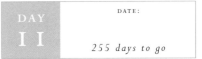

<table>
<tr><td>DAY
11</td><td>DATE:

255 days to go</td></tr>
</table>

Inside the hollow ball, a membrane forms that **divides it into two chambers**—one contains the empty yolk sac where the baby's intestines will form; the other is reserved for the developing baby. Soon some of the cells separate and form a thin membrane called the amnion, which surrounds both chambers.

About eight out of every ten women experience a classic symptom of pregnancy—**morning sickness**—as their bodies adjust to the increase in pregnancy-supporting hormones (estrogen, progesterone, and hCG) and changes in carbohydrate utilization. Nausea, with or without vomiting, can be provoked by sharp odors, especially fried foods, perfume, and cigarette smoke, and by ingesting processed foods, caffeine, and sweets. It also seems linked to low blood sugar—that's why women are urged to eat small meals every two hours, a snack at bedtime, and another before getting out of bed in the morning so that the stomach is never completely empty.

The surest way to make it hard for your children is to make it soft for them.
WESLEYAN METHODIST PROVERB

For Your Information The good news about the nausea and vomiting of pregnancy is that it generally reaches a peak in the third month (when hCG production peaks) and then declines noticeably in the fourth month. **The bad news is that morning sickness can occur at any time of the day or night.** Vitamin B$_6$ is often used to treat pregnancy-related nausea, and the symptoms usually disappear within a few hours. Check with your health practitioner regarding dosage.

Food Facts **Hardening of the baby's skeleton** by adding minerals to the cartilage to form bone will begin about six weeks from now and **won't be complete for 25 years!** Calcium, phosphorus, and vitamin K are needed to build the baby's bones and teeth. Vitamin D keeps calcium circulating in your bloodstream and aids the absorption of phosphorus. Vitamin C, copper, manganese, zinc, and fluoride are also involved. Each day, be sure to get at least 1,000 mg of calcium, 700 mg of phosphorus, 90 mcg of vitamin K, 200 IU (5 mcg) of vitamin D, 85 mg of vitamin C, 1,000 mcg of copper, 2 mg of manganese, and 11 mg of zinc. Fluoride can be supplemented up to 3 mg but most pregnant women drink fluoridated water.

DAY 12	DATE: 254 days to go

The embryo now looks like two hollow balls stacked like beads on a string. The bead closest to the placenta is attached to the implantation site by a short, thick umbilical cord. **Everything is encased by a fluid-filled bubble.** The bubble, of course, is the amniotic sac. Your embryonic baby measures between 0.006 and 0.008 inch in length (0.15 to 0.20 mm). **Five embryos could fit into the space occupied by this printed period.**

Chart your waist size and weight here and on page 181.

WAIST SIZE   WEIGHT

Fatigue, stress, and a prepregnancy diet low in vitamins, minerals, and carbohydrates can make your nausea more severe. Pregnant women tend to feel better if their stomachs are neither too full or too empty, so don't overeat or let yourself go hungry. Take your prenatal vitamins before bedtime with a snack or with a meal. To combat fatigue, nap and go to bed as early as you can; take advantage of rest time on buses, trains, or when carpooling; and get someone to watch your other children so you can rest.

Food Facts Carbohydrates provide fuel for living organisms. You may feel better if you eat **complex carbohydrates** like those found in beans, peas, brown rice, and whole grain breads, cereals, and pasta. Natural nut butters (nothing added) with toast or crackers and natural dairy products like cheese and milk can help prevent an upset stomach. The recommended carbohydrate intake is about 50 percent of the day's calories. **You need a minimum of 130 g of carbohydrates a day just to meet the energy needs of your brain! You need 175 daily grams of carbs now that you're pregnant.**

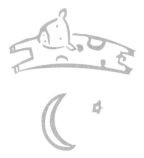

Your children are not your children. They are the sons and daughters of Life's longing for itself.
KAHLIL GIBRAN

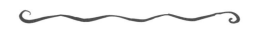

Did You Know? The first system to function in your developing baby is its heart and blood vessels. **Your baby's heart will be beating before your period is one week late!**

DAY 13	DATE: 253 days to go

Growth of the embryo continues to be rapid. Over the next two days, the tissue that lines the placenta appears. First-trimester **prenatal screening tests** are done to provide information about the baby's risk of having heart problems, Down syndrome, and other chromosomal disorders. They can involve a maternal blood test and an ultrasound exam. Discuss your options with your health-care provider.

If you need something to settle your stomach, ginger is a common Chinese remedy, but it may make your symptoms worse or encourage heartburn. Try sipping peppermint, spearmint, or lemon balm tea. Try pressing an accupressure point (pericardium point six) on your wrist, three finger widths from the point where your third finger is. Feel lightly for a slight dip and press dip quite deeply. You can buy wristbands which help you apply this pressure. Unfortunately, remedies that worked with your first pregnancy may not work with the second. Keep trying until you find something natural that works.

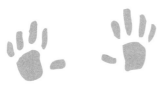

TIME TO REFLECT

When did you begin to think about having the baby?

_____

_____

_____

_____

Consider This A second pregnancy is typically suspected earlier and more accurately than the first. Odor sensitivity, nausea, fatigue, and sore gums may have a déjà vu quality if you've experienced all this before. If you know you're pregnant again because you can't stand the way things smell, for example, you will also anticipate that the other feelings and symptoms will start up again. . . . But it's different this time, even though it might seem the same. You're carrying an entirely different baby in an entirely changed body under an entirely different set of circumstances. **And for the sake of *this* baby, let yourself experience the wonder of this extraordinary time absolutely unjaded.**

Childbirth Then and Now In the second century CE, the Greek physician Galen proposed a theory of prenatal development called emboîtement, from a word meaning "encasement" or "encapsulation." He thought that tiny, preformed babies existed in the "female semen" and that contact with the male merely brought about an "unshelling" of the baby, permitting it to increase in size until birth.

When I approach a child, he inspires in me two sentiments:
tenderness for what he is, and respect for what he may become.
LOUIS PASTEUR

DAY **14**	DATE: _____
	252 days to go

The placenta is now fully lined. The amniotic sac, amniotic cavity, umbilical stalk, and yolk sac have also completed their development. **The cells that will form the baby have flattened into a structure called the embryonic disc.**

You may find that you are more tired than usual, especially if you've been pregnant before. **Your body needs extra rest now** because of all the internal activity connected with your pregnancy. Stay well hydrated, but separate liquids from solids—**drink fluids mainly between meals**. If you are having trouble getting fluids in, eat water-rich foods such as clear soups, broth, celery, and watermelon. Drink diluted 100 percent natural vegetable juice or clear fruit juices. Rest and good hydration can also help you avoid catching a cold or **the flu; viral infections of all types can hurt the baby. Handwashing is a must year-round!**

Did You Know? **Women in their childbearing years** need 600 mcg of folic acid every day. Through foods and/or supplements, **folic acid helps prevent birth defects by making sure the baby's spinal cord is completely sealed along the spine** and none of it seeps out. Some breakfast cereals and other grain products are enriched with 100 percent of the folic acid your body needs every day.

Food Facts **Phytonutrients** are biologically active compounds found in plant-derived foods, such as fruits (especially raspberries, blueberries, apples, and red and purple grapes), herbs, spices, walnuts, beans, peas, seeds, and vegetables (especially kale, spinach, and avocado). While there is no recommended daily intake of phytonutrients, there's no question that these compounds have the potential to help women, pregnant or otherwise, **stay healthy** and prevent disease. Be sure to include them in your diet.

What do you want to be sure to remember?

(See page 28 for more space to write.)

The childhood shows the man, as morning shows the day.

JOHN MILTON

LMP Week 5

DAY 15	DATE:
	251 days to go

The primitive streak appears (this is **the forerunner of the brain and spinal cord).** It is now possible to identify the head and tail sections of your baby's body.

By the end of this third week, you'll probably miss your menstrual period for the first time. You can celebrate your suspicions with a bottle of sparkling apple juice, grape juice, or ginger ale. **Even one alcoholic beverage, no matter how diluted, can cause birth defects.** When you drink, your baby drinks, too, and there is much more alcohol in their system than in yours because they are so tiny!

IMPORTANT: Worldwide, **alcohol use during pregnancy is the #1 known cause of preventable mental retardation in children.** In the United States, every container of beer, wine, or liquor sold warns women about the impact of alcohol on their developing babies. Your baby needs every advantage you can offer. Right now, exposure to alcohol would be a major disadvantage with potential complications. **If you find it difficult to go without, get help quitting.**

Did You Know? The implanted embryo can be detected by ultrasound as early as today.

DAY 16	DATE:
	250 days to go

The flat embryonic disc now has three distinct layers of tissue, each containing stem cells. **All of the baby's cells and organs will form from these three tissue layers.** Here are their contributions:

ENDODERM: thyroid, pancreas, liver, lining of lungs, tongue, tonsils, urethra, bladder, adrenal gland, stomach, and intestines.

MESODERM: all muscles, bones, immune system, spleen, red blood cells, heart, lungs, reproductive structures, and the systems that remove urine and sweat.

ECTODERM: skin pigment cells, nails, hair, lens of the eye, tissues associated with ear, nose, and sinuses, tongue (taste buds), mouth, anus, tooth enamel, pituitary glands, mammary glands, nervous system, and brain.

Pregnant women need 27 mg of **iron** each day. Eat foods rich in iron such as hormone-free lean red meat, chicken, sustainable fish, and fortified eggs. If you don't eat meat, other foods that contain iron include blackstrap molasses; whole-grain breads and pasta; iron-fortified cereal, quinoa, tofu, and organic oatmeal; and dried apricots and figs.

Food Facts **Cookware may have an effect on food during cooking.** Replace any pots, pans, or utensils with coating that can chip or slough off and release toxic chemicals. Bamboo paddles, wooden spoons, chopsticks, and crockery appear to have no harmful effects on food during cooking. In addition, bamboo and wood are renewable resources.

Many small make a great.
JOHN HEYWOOD

Unglazed cast iron increases levels of dietary iron. Cookware that is made of anodized aluminum, copper with stainless steel lining, stainless steel, and bamboo steamers are not reactive.

DAY 17	DATE:
	249 days to go

The cells involved in building the nervous system compress to form a groove called the notochord, which gives rise to the spinal cord and the discs of tissue between the bones of the spine. The cells at one end of the notochord release a chemical that causes rapid growth and the appearance of a thickened area called the neural plate. This plate will form the baby's head. Your baby is now 0.02 inch long (0.4 mm). **Two or three babies the size of yours could fit into the space occupied by this printed period.**

Avoiding viral illness during pregnancy is about more than just reducing your downtime. Viruses—those associated with measles, flu, rubella, and herpes (HSV) (just to name a few)—may transmit **an infection that disturbs your baby's brain development.** Ask your health-care provider about a flu shot and other ways to avoid viral infections.

Chart your waist size and weight here and on page 181.

WAIST SIZE   WEIGHT

IMPORTANT: These early weeks (Days 17 through 56) mark a **critical period in a baby's brain development.** Safeguarding development now and throughout pregnancy is key. Counting your newborn's fingers and toes tells you *nothing* about the integrity of his or her brain.

For Your Information **The impact of exposure to health hazards is always a function of each person's potential susceptibility.** Some individuals are relatively more sensitive and some are relatively less. Since it's impossible to tell how resistant you may (or may not) be to a potential hazard, you are always urged to err on the side of caution. Hazards to avoid include chemicals in pool and cleaning products, pesticides and herbicides, gasoline and petroleum products, smog, paint, and secondhand smoke from any source.

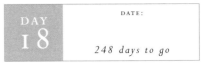

DAY 18	DATE:
	248 days to go

Besides forming the baby's first blood cells and vessels, the cells that create the blood islands also form channels called the heart tubes. The heart tubes are fusing together. **This marks the first step in forming a rough draft of the baby's heart** that will begin to circulate the blood cells throughout its body by the end of this week.

Most changes that accompany pregnancy are normal, and although they may be uncomfortable, they are no cause for alarm. However, some symptoms need to be reported as soon as they occur so your practitioner can determine their importance.

Contact your health-care provider *right away* if you experience vaginal bleeding, pelvic or lower abdominal pain, or persistent backache.

Children seldom misquote you. They more often repeat word for word what you shouldn't have said.
MAE MALOO

Food Facts While **fish and shellfish** contain heart- and brain-healthy omega-3 fatty acids, the oceans are polluted with mercury and other toxic chemicals. The U.S. Food and Drug Administration recommends limiting fish intake to 12 oz per week from safer, sustainable varieties that don't absorb as much mercury (avoid shark, swordfish, marlin, tilefish, or king mackerel). **Even low levels of toxins can harm a baby's developing brain and nervous system.** Clear guidelines for specifying fish as organic have been marked by disagreements over what organic fish should eat. Fish oil supplements are not recommended during pregnancy because too much vitamin A is toxic. Work with your healthcare provider to establish a safe fish intake plan that's right for you or get your omega-3s from another source.

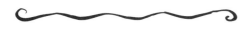

TIME TO REFLECT
When did you first suspect you were pregnant?

....
....
....
....
....

What do you want to be sure to remember?

....
....
....
....
....
....
....

(See page 28 for more space to write.)

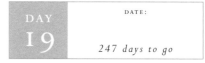

DAY 19	DATE:
	247 days to go

The tissue that will form the baby's head can now be identified and begins to fold inward around the notochord **to create your baby's brain.** The baby measures between 0.04 and 0.06 inch (1.0 to 1.5 mm) from head to tail, just big enough to rest on the point of a ballpoint pen.

Breast changes can be expected as your pregnancy continues. Tingling sensations and some soreness may be felt in your breasts during this early part of pregnancy.

For Your Health **Caffeine** crosses the placenta and is hard for the baby to metabolize; also, it may be **associated with low birth weight and miscarriage** because of uterine contractions. As a diuretic, it reduces the total amount of fluid in the woman's body, and larger quantities can cause nervousness, irritability, and sleep problems. Pregnant women are urged to avoid caffeine consumption. One cup of brewed coffee has four to five times more caffeine than one 12 oz cola beverage. The decaf versions of coffee, tea, and soda reduce caffeine by about 97 percent.

Food Facts **Heavy processing leaves food with little nutrient value.** Eat cleaner, fresh foods that are freer from chemical add-ons—artificial sweeteners, refined sugars, artificial flavoring, artificial colors, preservatives, hormones, pesticides, and high levels of salt and fat. Evaluate the list of ingredients and nutrition facts before you buy heat-and-eat products (such as frozen meals) and ready-to-eat products (such as commercial salad or frozen ice cream treats). Choose food from chain restaurants with great care.

What's done to children, they will do to society.
KARL MENNINGER

DAY	DATE:
20	*246 days to go*

For the **next 30 days, a critical period in the development of baby's heart** will overlap with the intense growth of the muscles, brain, spinal cord, and nervous system. While the heart itself consists of just two heart tubes, it must join with the blood vessels that have been forming within your baby's chest. As the circulatory system pieces itself together, the tissue on either side of the spinal cord begins dividing into blocks of cells called *somites*. Somites eventually form the bones and muscles of your baby's head and body. Today, the first pair of somites will appear, and 38 pairs will eventually form between now and Day 30. Elsewhere in the body, the thyroid glands, eventually located at the base of the neck on either side of the windpipe, are also beginning to form. Today is a big day in the development of your baby's muscles, bones, spinal cord, and heart.

Calcium, magnesium, and potassium are nutrients that **directly affect the development of the baby's heart.** Calcium and potassium regulate the rhythm of the heart by helping its muscle contract, while magnesium relaxes muscles in general and helps prevent preterm labor. Almost all the calcium and magnesium in the body is found in combination with phosphates. Make sure you get 1,000 mg of calcium, 4,700 mg of potassium, 360 mg of magnesium, and 700 mg of phosphorus daily.

Food Facts Again, **superfoods are the most nutritious natural foods you can eat.** These include dark-colored fruits (blueberries and strawberries, for example) and dark-colored vegetables such as kale and broccoli. Orange-colored vegetables like sweet potatoes and butternut squash are high in antioxidants that support overall health. However, just because these foods are good for you doesn't mean you should eat unlimited amounts.

DAY	DATE:
21	*245 days to go*

The primitive heart tubes are folded, remodeled, and divided to form a four-chambered heart. Three pairs of somites are now present along the spinal column. The tissue that will form the baby's eyes has already been reserved. The cavities of the chest and abdomen are forming. **Your baby** now measures about ⅛ inch (1.5 to 2.5 mm) and **is about the size of a sesame seed.**

The National Institutes of Health (NIH) recommends that pregnant women eat a total of 2,400 to 2,500 calories every day from healthy, high-quality sources—just about 300 additional calories per day. (The recommended daily intake for non-pregnant women is 2,100–2,300 cal.) **Low-calorie diets** can deprive the developing baby of the proteins, vitamins, and minerals needed for normal growth. Without proper nutrition, the woman's body will start to break down stored fat. Substances called ketones are a by-product of this process and, if left to accumulate, can **dull the development of baby's brain.**

Did You Know? By the fourth week, **the placenta** efficiently conducts nutrient, oxygen, and waste exchange between the mother and the baby. The placenta will also prepare your breasts for milk production (lactation).

For Your Information As important as good nutrition is during pregnancy, it's often easier not to eat right if this is your second pregnancy. Life is more hectic this time. Since you don't have as much time to shop or spend preparing food, you might find yourself relying more on fast food or takeout. And you may already have a fussy eater who likes only certain foods, making variety more of a challenge and mealtime more frustrating.

Pregnancy defined is: Getting company inside one's skin.

MAGGIE SCARF

Week 4 Begins

DAY 22	DATE:
	244 days to go

Between Week 4 and Week 8, the development of your baby's facial features takes place. By Day 28 or 30, four folds of tissue at the base of the head will provide the raw material for the chin, cheeks, upper and lower jaw, palate, mouth, tongue, neck, ears, and some of the nerves that control them. Right now, two such folds are present. Five more pairs of somites have formed. Now eight pairs of somites are present, and begin to surround the rough draft of the spinal cord. The chest and abdominal cavities are continuing to form. The urogenital ridge is formed, which will give rise to the urinary and reproductive structures. Lung buds (tissue from which the lungs will form) appear in the chest cavity.

Although you've been waiting for your period to start, **by now you probably have an idea that you might be pregnant.** A pregnancy test is always a good place to begin. Either check in with your clinic or physician or purchase a home pregnancy test kit. After a positive test, decide on a practitioner and schedule your first prenatal visit.

Did You Know? Circulation is beginning to develop in the lining of the placenta as the tiny muscles of your **baby's heart begin to beat sometime today.** The heart measures only 0.1 inch (2 mm) long. This seems impossibly small, but in proportion to the baby's body, your baby's heart is nine times as large as an adult's heart.

Food Facts **Water is involved in every aspect of your pregnancy.** Your baby floats in amniotic fluid that is replaced every three hours, and you're supporting 50 percent more blood volume—these are just two of the conspicuous examples of the high water demands of your body. Your goal is to consume 13 cups (3 liters) of clean water per day. Carry water with you wherever you go and sip it all day between meals (this will help you gauge your consumption). If you want something different, try a flavored water, tonic water, or anything with no sugar, no caffeine, and a little fizz. If it's cold where you live, substitute warm versions of the above.

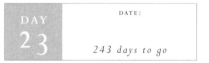

DAY 23	DATE:
	243 days to go

Development that began yesterday continues today: Your baby's jaws are appearing, the lung buds are forming, circulation is being established in the yolk sac, the lining of the placenta is developing, and four more pairs of somites have formed, bringing the total to 12 pairs. Right now, stem cells are migrating from the yolk sac to the back wall of the baby's body, where they will form the reproductive tract.

While you may be craving certain foods, **food cravings and aversions** are usually due to changes in taste and smell sensitivities and are unrelated to real physiological needs. A woman who craves pickles or chips is not likely to need salt in her diet, for example. You may also find that some things you eat disagree with you. Heartburn, indigestion, bloating, and other discomforts are not

---

Kids are confused. Half of the adults tell him to find himself; the other half tell him to get lost.

WALTER MACPEEK

uncommon during pregnancy. Identify the foods that tend to cause you digestive problems and avoid them as much as possible until you feel more stable.

Chart your waist size and weight here and on page 181.

WAIST SIZE   WEIGHT

For Your Health In addition to phytonutrients, **vegetable superfoods contain bioflavonoids.** Bioflavonoids are plant chemicals that help reduce inflammation, repair tissue, and promote healing. They may help reduce the risk of heart disease, cancer, diabetes, vision cell degeneration, autoimmune disorders like lupus, and premature aging and minimize the impact of environmental toxins like smog and secondhand tobacco smoke.

Did You Know? As long as you remain healthy, your kidneys can process 15 liters of water per day, so 13 cups (3 liters) is a piece of cake!

IMPORTANT: Cigarette smoking during pregnancy is the number one cause of preventable learning disabilities in children. If you need help to quit, get it now.

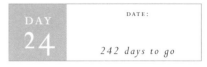

DATE:

DAY
24

242 days to go

The next 32 days (Days 24 through 56) mark a **critical period for arm and leg development.** At this point, your baby has no visible arms or legs, but within a few hours, the tiny buds that form the arms will suddenly appear. Sixteen pairs of somites are now present with the spinal cord forming in between. Liver and pancreas buds are also present. Incredibly, the opposite edges of the cell layers pull themselves together to form three concentric tubes of tissue. This folding process makes the embryo rounded rather than angular and curved rather than straight.

You may have noticed that you're **experiencing some of the same emotions that often precede menstruation**: moodiness, irritability, tearfulness. While some of these feelings may have a psychological basis, most of the time they are just natural reactions to your body's changing levels of hormones and can be amplified by your immediate experience.

Food Facts Pregnant women can consume more **phytochemicals** by eating more fruit; doubling the normal serving size of vegetables to 1 cup; using fresh herbs and spices in cooking, especially parsley, basil, hot peppers, and oregano; replacing some of the meat in their diet with whole grains, legumes, and vegetables (including radishes, cucumbers, endive, cabbage, and onions); adding grated vegetables to other foods, such as carrots to chili or meatballs, or celery and squash to spaghetti.

Childbirth is more admirable than conquest, more amazing than self-defense, and as courageous as either one.
GLORIA STEINEM

Did You Know? By the end of this month, your baby will have completed a period of growth that involves **the greatest size and physical changes of its lifetime.** In five days, it will be 10,000 times larger than the fertilized egg though, in actuality, not much bigger than a grain of rice!

Food Facts Cold ready-to-eat cereals made from whole grains (like oats, wheat, and corn) are valuable sources of B vitamins. Hot whole-grain cereals are also nutritious and rich in fiber—three times as much as in cold cereals. Check the **sugar and fat content** of all cereals carefully.

Can You Believe It? Your baby's heart is actually beating!

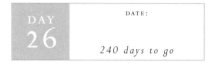

DAY 26

DATE:

240 days to go

The baby's body now has **a curved shape**, with a **prominent bump** representing his or her head, a **temporary tail-like structure**, and tiny bumps (called "buds") where your **baby's arms and legs** will be present. Your baby's length is now measured from the top of his or her head (crown) to the bottom of his or her bottom (rump). The **crown-to-rump length** at Day 26 is between 0.11 and 0.20 inch (3 to 5 mm)—a size that can easily fit on the eraser end of a standard lead pencil!

DAY 25

DATE:

241 days to go

The aorta, a large artery that carries blood away from the heart to all organs and tissues, is now forming. In addition, the tissue that will form your **baby's eyes** is present, and a tiny dimple now marks the place on either side of the head where the baby's ear canal and inner ear will form. Either today or tomorrow, **the top end of the tube that forms around the spinal cord closes to protect it.**

You may begin to notice a need to urinate more frequently. This is normal and due to an improved metabolism that eliminates waste more quickly. When you're farther along, your bladder will feel pressure from an enlarging uterus, and you'll again feel an increased need to urinate. Your breasts may feel fuller, heavier, and tender. You may also notice the areola, or pigmented portion of your breast, darkening somewhat.

IMPORTANT: This week marks a critical period in the development of your baby's digestive system—his or her **intestines are beginning to form** from a portion of the yolk sac.

Selecting a practitioner is an extremely important task. You need to weigh many considerations as you choose the person who will direct the medical course of your pregnancy and attend the birth of your baby. A referral from a trusted person is a good place to start but not always available. You'll want to know about their philosophy of childbirth: Will they consult with you? How do they help the laboring woman manage pain? Will they attend a home birth if that is an option? And so on.

For Your Information **The stomach is such an important organ** that a slight swelling in your baby's developing gut already marks its appearance.

I think that saving the little child and bringing him to his own, /
Is a derned site better business than loafing around the throne.

JOHN HEY

Did You Know? The **baby's tiny heart** pumps 65 times a minute to circulate the newly formed blood cells and nourish developing tissues.

TIME TO REFLECT

When your pregnancy was confirmed, how did you react?

....

....

....

....

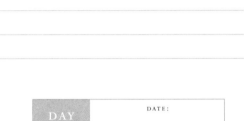

DAY 27	DATE:
	239 days to go

By now a tiny **liver** has formed. The liver plays an important role in the utilization of nutrients: It stores excess blood sugar and releases it when required, it stores and breaks down fat, it breaks down excess protein, it produces blood-clotting factors, and it breaks down toxic substances like alcohol. **The gall bladder, stomach, intestines, pancreas, and lungs are also beginning to form.**

During your **first prenatal visit**, your practitioner will take a complete history of your general and reproductive health, estimate a due date, identify any pregnancy-related risk factors, run some tests, suggest healthy habits, provide information about screening and diagnostic tests, and give you a preview of what lies ahead.

IMPORTANT: If your baby's heart didn't begin to beat yesterday, it will start today. However, **it will take a few more days for the heartbeat to be strong enough to be detected by Doppler technology.**

Food Facts **Fat** is necessary for good health. Begin a diet that benefits both you and your baby by eating fats that protect the heart and brain from deposits of clogging plaques. The most nutritious sources of fats are in plant foods and in fish that eat microscopic plants. Since **your body cannot make these essential omega-3 and omega-6 fatty acids in sufficient quantities to meet your or your baby's needs (no one's can, pregnant or not), these must be supplied by diet.** Healthy plant sources of fat include avocados; olives; nuts and nut butters (including soy); tofu; some seeds (sesame, flaxseed, pumpkin, sunflower); and vegetable oils (safflower, olive). Healthy omega fat from fish comes from wild salmon, farm-raised catfish and trout, sardines, and shrimp. (Remember that all natural fish and shellfish can contain some mercury and contaminants.)

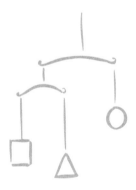

Where did you come from baby dear? Out of the everywhere into the here.

GEORGE MACDONALD

<table>
<tr><td>DAY
28</td><td>DATE:

238 days to go</td></tr>
</table>

A tiny depression on either side of your baby's head marks the location where the eyes are forming. The arm buds appear as swellings on the side of the baby's body; the leg buds will be more visible in another day or two. The first of three sets of kidneys appear. (This set never becomes functional, however.) **The baby is shaped like a C**, and the tail portion becomes less prominent as body growth catches up to spinal cord growth.

Today marks the end of the first month of your pregnancy (each gestational month is based on a lunar month of 28 days, or four 7-day weeks). Only 8½ more months to go!

Did You Know? Now that you're pregnant you're not really "eating for two." You only **need 300 more healthy calories per day, but up to 100 percent more various nutrients than do nonpregnant women.** Keep in mind that you're not "getting fat"—you're building your baby's body and brain!

Food Facts **Just as there are heart- and brain-healthy fats, there are also unhealthy ones.** Saturated fats are solid at room temperature and come from fatty meats like beefsteak, poultry skin and wings, dairy products like ice cream, and lard. Trans fats are chemically altered saturated oils that become solid at room temperature, and behave like solid fats in the body. They are found in processed foods, baked goods like cakes and pastries, fried foods like French fries and donuts, crackers, and other snack foods. All of these "bad" fats can lower the level of "good" blood cholesterol (HDL) which moves dangerous (LDL) cholesterol out of the body. In addition, unhealthy fat can build up inside of the blood vessels, reduce blood flow, and coat brain cells with Alzheimer's-like plaques.

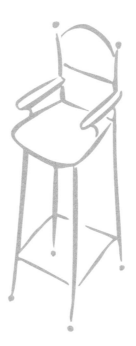

What do you want to remember about your **First Month?**

Lunar Month 2

THINGS TO DO THIS MONTH:

* Eat sufficient folic acid and vitamins C and B_{12}, all of which are critical for supporting the baby's developing brain.

* Take sufficient vitamin D, which significantly reduces the likelihood of preeclampsia.

* Get sufficient dietary fiber.

* Don't smoke tobacco or marijuana, drink alcohol, or use illegal drugs.

* Check with your healthcare provider about being exposed to essential oils and aromatic blends.

* Do Kegel exercises.

* Drink lots of water between meals.

* Discuss troublesome mood swings with your practitioner.

* Don't use acne medicine.

* Moisturize your skin; keep oily skin clean.

* If you want chocolate, eat raw chocolate or raw, unprocessed cocoa. Check for caffeine in other chocolate products.

* Avoid or reduce the symptoms of acid indigestion by eliminating coffee, carbonated drinks, caffeine, citrus, and milk.

* Wash your hands frequently or use alcohol-free hand sanitizers; have your children do the same.

Week 5 Begins

DAY 29	DATE: 237 days to go

The body gives special attention to the development of the nerve that takes visual images to the brain, the cells that transmit those images, and the lens of **each eye.** The lens bends the light that enters the eye to focus a clear image for interpretation. Elsewhere, the surface layer of **baby's skin** will be formed during this month; the **tongue** is recognizable; the **nasal pits** are beginning to form; the **immune system**, which filters out bacteria and other foreign particles, is beginning to develop; a second nonfunctional set of kidneys appears; the **arms** look like flippers; and **leg buds are visible.** At five weeks, the baby's body cavity contains all the tissues needed to develop the baby's **reproductive structures**, beginning with the ovaries (if your baby is a girl) or testes (if your baby is a boy). Whew!

During the next six days, the **baby's brain, body, and head will undergo a period of particularly rapid growth.** The head grows faster than other organs, mostly because of the rapid development of the brain and face. Do all you can to support this growth. **Folic acid and vitamins C and B$_{12}$** are crucial. Spinach, turnip greens, lettuces, asparagus, broccoli, oranges, cantaloupe, strawberries, garbanzo beans or chickpeas, and pinto beans are all natural sources of folic acid. Choose fresh organically grown foods if possible. Bring on the freshly-made hummus!

Did You Know? Leg development always lags slightly behind arm development until the third year of your baby's life.

Food Facts **Vitamins must be obtained from foods or supplements because they cannot be synthesized by our cells.** As little as 5 to 15 minutes of sunlight exposure two to three times a week on the hands, face, and arms helps our skin produce vitamin D. Vitamin D is an essential nutrient that strengthens bones by helping with the absorption of calcium and activates the immune system to prevent illness. Very few natural foods contain vitamin D. Dietary sources of vitamin D include eggs, fortified milk and orange juice, fish, and cod liver oil. Check with your health-care provider regarding dosage; most supplements contain 200 IU.

IMPORTANT: Women who **take the recommended dose of vitamin D** during pregnancy are five times less likely to develop the dangerously fluctuating blood pressure levels characteristic of preeclampsia. Preeclampsia is the number one cause of maternal and fetal mortality.

Chart your waist size and weight here and on page 181.

WAIST SIZE	WEIGHT

DAY 30	DATE: 236 days to go

By this time, 38 pairs of *somites* (blocks of cells that form the bones and muscles of the head and trunk) have formed. If they haven't appeared already, the leg buds will be present today. **Your baby's brain has organized into the three main parts possessed by all human**

There are only two things a child will share willingly—communicable diseases and his mother's age.

DR. BENJAMIN SPOCK

brains: the forebrain, the midbrain, and the hindbrain. The hindbrain contains regions that help regulate heart rate and breathing and coordinate muscle movement; the midbrain is a relay station (routes "messages" to their final destinations in the brain) and contains emotion centers; and the forebrain has specialized structures called lobes that translate input from the senses, play a role in memory formation and storage, and engage in higher-order processing like thinking, reasoning, and problem solving. Your baby is about ⅓ inch (5 to 7 mm) long—about the size of a half of an M&M—that's **15,000 times bigger than at conception in only 30 days.** And that's not all! In just one week (by Day 37), your baby will be twice as long as he or she is today.

An ultrasound test or sonogram can be performed any time from this point (Week 5) on to **estimate the date of conception by measuring the baby's crown-to-rump length.** This measurement is accurate to between one and four days of development. Because the somites are so prominent, they are also used to determine the embryo's age. Your practitioner will discuss the rationale behind any prenatal diagnostic procedures ordered.

Did You Know? The yolk sac that developed early in the first month is now nonfunctional and will diminish in size. It remains a tiny lump of useless tissue until birth, when it is expelled as part of the afterbirth.

Food Facts **Eggs from healthy chickens** are a balanced source of all important vitamins (except vitamin C) and minerals and may be enriched with nutrients like omega-3 fatty acids, for example. Each egg offers about 6 g of high-quality protein.

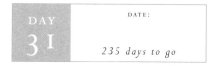

Rapid brain growth continues. By this time, the tube that protects the spinal cord has usually closed. The hypothalamus—a structure critical to the regulation of thirst, eating, sexual behavior, and body temperature—begins to form today or tomorrow. Cups are formed that will cradle the eyeballs, a rough draft of the mouth appears, and the *larynx* (voice box) has begun to develop. No skull plates are in place yet. The groove of tissue that appeared on Day 22 will now separate from the *trachea* (windpipe) and will develop into the *esophagus* (the tube through which food is swallowed).

Most women don't notice much change in their own bodies yet. When your pregnancy first starts to show, the baby bump will appear in **your lower abdomen beneath your belly button.** That's where your uterus is.

For Your Information It takes five weeks (from Week 4 through Week 8) for the main organs and systems in the baby's body to get their start. In the next two days, ribs will begin to project from the tiny backbone to protect the developing organs in the chest. And **by the end of this month, the embryo in your womb will look like a tiny baby!**

Food Facts **Natural soybeans** are the only food in the vegetable kingdom that contains all the essential amino acids the body needs to synthesize protein. Soy foods are an excellent source of protein and are high in calcium, iron, zinc, thiamin, B_6, folate, and vitamin E, and are also a source of omega-3 fatty acids. However, soy also contains a chemical that mimics estrogen, a female hormone that can affect your baby's development. Discuss the use of natural soy and soy-containing products with your practitioner.

Once you bring life into this world, you must protect it. We must protect it by changing the world.
ELIE WEISEL

<table>
<tr><td>DAY
32</td><td>DATE:

234 days to go</td></tr>
</table>

Your baby's arms now look less like flippers and more like paddles. The muscles that will surround the bones of your **baby's arms and legs** begin to migrate into those regions sometime this week. Nerves also grow into the developing limbs. The mouth looks large in relation to baby's clearly defined jaws. And, in about nine days, the tissue that forms the **tongue muscle** will have migrated into the region where the face is forming. Muscles on a mission!

Dietary fiber helps relieve constipation and move solid waste out of your system (it moves the baby's waste, too). A diet high in fiber helps you maintain healthy cholesterol and blood-sugar levels. It also helps prevent bowel cancer by keeping waste moving and preventing blockage. During pregnancy, 28 g of fiber per day is recommended.

For Your Health The recommended **salt** intake for a regular diet is about 3,000 mg per day—the equivalent of ½ teaspoon of table salt. Pregnancy is a condition that actually requires more salt. The extra sodium is needed to regulate water use and distribution in a system processing much more fluid than usual. However, sometimes there are medical reasons to restrict salt intake during pregnancy. The healthiest salt is unrefined; processed food often contains a huge amount of processed salt.

Did You Know? **Amniotic fluid** is manufactured by the baby. First, it is secreted through the baby's skin before the surface layer of the skin is formed. Amniotic fluid is also secreted by the baby's lungs at a rate of 1¼ to 1¾ cups (300 to 400 ml) daily.

Food Facts **Organic dairy milk** is an excellent source of protein, calcium, phosphorus, vitamin A, and vitamin D. Again, during pregnancy, your body needs 200 IU of vitamin D daily to promote the absorption of calcium by your intestine. (The calcium in soy milk is less bioavailable than from organic cow's milk.) Low-fat milk is probably the best choice during pregnancy to avoid excess fat and calories; however, whole milk or lactase-treated milk is sometimes better tolerated.

<table>
<tr><td>DAY
33</td><td>DATE:

233 days to go</td></tr>
</table>

The pits that will become the nostrils are now prominent. The developing heart can be seen through your baby's chest wall. The final (and permanent) set of kidneys has been formed. And in about a week, the kidneys will produce urine. In the next four days the hand plates will appear. Each round hand plate contains the tissues that will form the palms and fingers. Your baby now measures about ⅜ inch (7 to 9 mm) in length. **Two babies the size of yours could fit on the surface of an American dime.**

Take 1.4 mg of vitamin B_1 (thiamin) and 6 mg of vitamin B_5 (pantothenic acid) daily. **These vitamins help release the energy from foods containing carbohydrates.** Thiamin also helps promote normal appetite and is essential for the development of your baby's brain, nervous system, and heart, as well as the liver, kidneys, and skeletal muscles.

Food Facts Eco-friendly wheat germ, ham, oysters, peanuts, green peas, and raisins are rich natural sources of thiamin; beef, chicken, whole grains, potatoes, tomatoes, broccoli, and mushrooms contain **vitamin B_5, which can be destroyed by processing, canning, or freezing foods.**

Kids really brighten a household. They never turn off the lights.
RALPH BUS

IMPORTANT: Most women who drink alcohol either consistently, excessively, or in binges become deficient in B vitamins, particularly thiamin and folic acid, and may also get less protein and magnesium than they need. Since these are essential nutrients, you can see why **drinking alcohol during pregnancy puts the baby at risk for brain damage and mental retardation.** After birth, alcohol easily enters the breast milk and can overwhelm the baby's system.

What do you want to be sure to remember?

(See page 48 for more space to write.)

DAY	DATE:
34	*232 days to go*

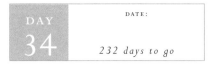
Because of the rapid brain growth that has been occurring, **your baby's head is much larger than his or her trunk.** The location of baby's nose is easily seen, and the muscles that control the baby's eyes are forming. Your baby's legs now resemble paddles. Soon, 42 to 44 somites will be present.

You will continue to **feel more tired** than usual. Rest when you're tired; try not to push yourself, since exhaustion comes more rapidly than before. If you're on a schedule and worried that you'll sleep too long, use an easy-to-set alarm clock.

IMPORTANT: Essential oils used for massage and aromatic blends can be put in a vaporizer and inhaled. Just like drugs and medicines, these chemicals can cross the placenta and affect your baby's development. **Given the uncertainty of their impact, it's best to avoid using essential oils and aromatherapy during pregnancy.**

DAY	DATE:
35	*231 days to go*

By now, the division between baby's **right brain and left brain** is well marked. The upper and lower jaws are present. Mammary gland tissue is beginning to develop into breasts in both females and males. Like in other mammals, nipples or breasts may form anywhere along the mammary ridge that extends from baby's underarms to the tops of the thighs.

Your ovaries don't ovulate during pregnancy. Many immature egg cells on the surface of the ovary temporarily develop, but never to the point of maturity because the hormones are balanced to favor the baby's development. Today marks the end of the fifth week of your pregnancy.

Did You Know? By this time, your embryonic baby displays a whole-body reflex in response to touch. This means that the **baby's developing nervous system is communicating with the young**

In their eagerness for their children to acquire skills and to succeed, parents may forget that youngsters need time to think, and privacy in which to do it.

JAMES COX

muscles, and the muscles are beginning to respond automatically to the system's commands. *All* of your baby's behavior, both in your uterus and after birth, originates from the basic capacity to form reflex responses.

For Your Information Your baby weighs about 0.00004 oz (0.001 g)—that's **about as heavy as an eyelash** from your lower lid.

Food Facts **Vitamin B$_2$ (riboflavin)** helps the body capture and use the energy released from carbohydrates, proteins, and fats. Riboflavin promotes tissue growth and repair, and normal vision. It is **critical to all tissues**, and very little of it is stored in the body. During pregnancy, 1.4 mg is required daily. One cup of 2 percent milk supplies one-third of the minimum daily riboflavin requirement.

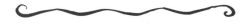

TIME TO REFLECT
How long did it take to become pregnant? Did it seem quick or slow?

What do you want to be sure to remember?

(See page 48 for more space to write.)

Children are travelers newly arrived in a strange country; we should therefore make conscience not to mislead them.
JOHN LOCKE

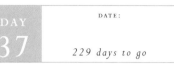

LMP Week 8

DAY **36**	DATE: _____ 230 days to go

The area of the **brain** that coordinates muscle movement (cerebellum) is beginning to develop. A rough draft of the **palate** is forming on the roof of your baby's mouth. Your baby's **hand plates** will appear by today if they aren't already present. The **elbow and wrist** regions of the arm are becoming identifiable. The **spleen** (the organ that produces antibodies and removes worn-out red blood cells and bacteria from the bloodstream) can be seen. By Week 9 the bulging **liver** makes up about 10 percent of your baby's body weight and produces red blood cells.

You'll want to ask your health-care provider about **Kegel exercises** to strengthen the muscles of your pelvic floor. When these muscles and the muscles in your back are properly toned, they will help carry the heavy uterus, help stop and start the flow of urine, and be more responsive during labor and delivery.

Food Facts **Avoid fatty processed breakfast meats** during pregnancy. Pork sausage, bacon, and breakfast sausage may contain as much as 50 percent fat and are highly processed. Breakfast meats made from turkey are leaner, but there are healthier sources of protein for breakfast—whole grains like steel-cut oatmeal and omega-3 enriched eggs, for example.

Childbirth in Other Cultures In ancient Japan, the umbilical cord was severed from the placenta after birth and wrapped in several thicknesses of white paper, with the outer covering containing the full names of the mother and the father. Once the child became an adult, the paper-wrapped cord was carried with them constantly.

DAY **37**	DATE: _____ 229 days to go

The **pituitary**, or master gland, is beginning to form in your baby's brain. This gland produces growth hormone and other hormones that regulate the function of the thyroid, adrenal glands (on top of the kidneys), and gonads (ovaries or testes). The olfactory bulb (connected with the **sense of smell**) is also beginning to form in the brain. During the next four days, pigment will begin to form in the **eyes**, making them easy to spot, and the lower limbs will develop **foot plates.** The **windpipe** (trachea), **voice box** (larynx), tubes that lead to the lungs (**bronchi**), and **tooth buds** for the baby teeth are forming. Your baby now measures 0.3 to 0.43 inch long (8 to 11 mm), having **doubled in length in just eight short days.** Now one baby the size of yours can fit within the perimeter of a dime.

Like riboflavin, **niacin** (vitamin B$_3$) helps your body capture and use the energy released from carbohydrates, proteins, and fats. It is of critical importance to all tissues, especially your baby's brain, nervous system, and liver.

Did You Know? **Your baby is growing at a phenomenal rate.** If your child grew as fast right after birth as it is growing right now, it would measure 15 feet tall by the time he or she was one month old!

Food Facts **Daily niacin** intake during pregnancy should be 18 mg, but niacin levels are usually adequate if protein intake is adequate. Niacin-rich sources include natural peanuts, the white meat of hormone-free chicken, and tuna canned in water. Supplementation during pregnancy may not be recommended.

DAY 38	DATE:
	228 days to go

Swellings are developing where the external **ears** will eventually be. The upper lip is beginning to form. The **intestines** are continuing to form within the umbilical cord. The shortage of space within baby's gut is due to the massive liver and two sets of kidneys. The cells that will produce your baby's **eggs or sperm** actually form in the yolk sac and then migrate to the pelvis in a day or two.

No matter how happy you are to be having a baby, you may experience some degree of **irritability or depression. Mood changes— especially significant ones—alter the chemical environment of your body and can influence baby's tendency toward fussiness and agitation.** Your first line of defense—*breathe*! Ten long, slow breaths—in through your nose, out through your mouth. Sit if you can. Close your eyes. Clear your mind and listen to the air entering and leaving your body. Do this every time you feel tension coming on.

Food Facts **Vitamin B$_{12}$** plays a role in protecting nerve fibers, promoting nervous system growth, and producing red blood cells. A daily intake of 2.6 mcg of vitamin B$_{12}$ is recommended during pregnancy. Anyone who eats meat, eggs, or milk products on a daily basis is guaranteed an adequate intake. Strict vegetarians can supplement their diets or drink vitamin B$_{12}$–fortified soy milk.

Did You Know? As you read about your baby's progress, perhaps you've noticed that the arms develop before the legs, the upper lip forms before the lower lip, and the brain grows more sophisticated than the rest of the organs. There is a pattern here:

for some cell clusters, growth proceeds from the head to the tail. Thus, organs and systems have to wait their respective turns, since some development is sequential rather than random or simultaneous.

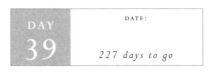

DAY 39	DATE:
	227 days to go

By tomorrow, your baby's lower limb paddles will have developed **foot plates** and pigment will be present in your **baby's eyes**. Several small swellings, which will become the **ear canal** and the **grooves of the outer ear**, are present on each side of baby's head.

Your skin may start to break out or dry out. **Complexion problems** are due to an increased secretion of oils and to the hormonal changes of pregnancy. Keep your skin clean, but ask your practitioner's advice on product safety.

Do not take acne medication or use topical acne medications because they both enter your bloodstream and can affect your baby.

For Your Comfort Moisturize dry skin. Ask your practitioner about rashes and skin that itches. Skin tags may also develop. These are little pieces of hanging skin. If you're bothered by them, see your dermatologist.

Food Facts **Cacao** (raw chocolate) and **raw, unprocessed cocoa** are superfoods with more than 300 chemically identifiable compounds, phytonutrients, and bioflavonoids. Some of these compounds work with our systems to elevate mood, keep us alert, help maintain healthy blood flow and blood pressure, and increase sensitivity to insulin (which protects against diabetes). They have the highest antioxidant value of any natural food in the world (Oxygen

There is only one pretty child in the world, and every mother has it.

OLD ENGLISH PROVERB

Radical Absorbance Capacity score of 28,000, with manufactured dark chocolate at 13,120 and manufactured milk chocolate at 6,740). **Antioxidants improve the lifespan of functioning cells.** Chocolate may have added caffeine, however. One ounce—a 28 g piece of bittersweet/dark chocolate—contains about 34 mg of caffeine compared to 95 to 200 mg in a cup of brewed coffee. Caffeine is hidden in other foods and beverages as well. Be sure to check labels carefully.

IMPORTANT: If you can't abstain, try to **limit your caffeine intake** to the equivalent of 1 cup of coffee per day or less.

DAY 40	DATE:
	226 days to go

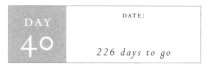 The **palate** continues to develop. The baby's **eyes** look pigmented (eye color won't be established until after birth). The jaw and facial muscles are beginning to form, but the eye muscles complete their development tomorrow. The **baby teeth** (or first teeth) are developing beneath your baby's gums. The baby's **heart** begins to mature its four chambers. **At this time, the heart's energy output is 20 percent that of an adult.** The **body cavity divides itself** into one segment that will contain the heart and lungs and another that will house the organs of the abdomen.

Hot whole-grain cereals provide more than just fiber; they also contain important B vitamins, minerals, and phytonutrients. Most hot cereals made from natural ingredients are low in fat, but check for sugar and additives just the same. Quaker Instant Oatmeal is 30 to 40 percent sugar.

Did You Know? During these first 40 days of development, your baby has grown 0.04 inch (1 mm) a day, but the **growth rate** is not even throughout its body: one day, growth may be concentrated in the arms, the next day, in the back, and so forth.

Food Facts Since your baby's teeth (and bones) require calcium for their development, you may be surprised to learn that **some vegetables and other foods are richer in calcium than milk, cheese, or yogurt.** That list includes arugula (1,300 mg per 100 calories), watercress (800 mg per 100 calories), turnip greens, collard greens, mustard greens (dark-green, leafy vegetables), broccoli, dried beans and peas, nuts and seeds, tofu, and sardines. Select your nutrients from natural sources.

DAY 41	DATE:
	225 days to go

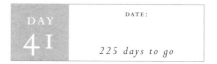 Because of all the rapid development, your **baby's head is now much larger than its trunk** and bent over a bump of tissue that contains the developing heart. Over the next two days, the neck and trunk will begin to straighten (remember, prior to this point, your embryonic baby has been shaped like a C). Also, within the next two days, the hand plates will develop ridges indicating where your baby's fingers and thumbs will be. As the process of forming these digital ridges continues, the baby's hands will look like the fan-shaped shell of a scallop. Your baby now measures nearly ½ inch long (11 to 14 mm). Baby is so small he or she would fit into a peanut shell, and weighs less than the whole peanut in that shell.

It is dangerous to confuse children with angels.
SIR DAVID MAXWELL FYFE

Vitamin B$_6$ helps your body use protein to build tissue and red blood cells. It's important to the immune system, helps support the organs that make white blood cells, and stabilizes the amount of glucose in the bloodstream. As you might suspect, your body needs almost 50 percent more B$_6$ during pregnancy in order to build your baby—1.9 mg daily. The best food sources include tuna, turkey, beef, chicken, salmon, sweet potato, sunflower seeds, spinach, and banana.

Chart your waist size and weight here and on page 181.

WAIST SIZE   WEIGHT

Food Facts One cup of ready-to-eat 100 percent B$_6$-fortified cereal supplies a full day's supply of the vitamin. Outside of that, a baked potato (with skin), raw banana, garbanzo beans, chicken breast, and lean pork are the richest natural sources of **vitamin B$_6$.** Make sustainable choices.

IMPORTANT: The body can't store more than a month's supply of vitamin B$_6$, so dietary sources are important. Supplemental vitamin B$_6$, niacin, and vitamin C should not be taken in excessive amounts. **Check upper limits with your practitioner.**

Childbirth in Other Cultures Historically, certain Filipino tribes believed that eating twin bananas could cause twins and that eating eggplant could cause a baby to be born with dark skin.

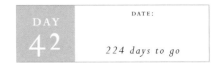

DAY 42	DATE:
	224 days to go

The digital ridges of the hand plates should be completed today. Within the heart, the blood vessel that sends blood to the lungs to gather oxygen (pulmonary artery) separates from the aorta. **Your baby's kidneys are beginning to produce urine** as they start their ascent to their final position near the small of the back. Today, the

One of the obvious facts about grown-ups to a child is that they have forgotten what it is like to be a child.
RANDALL JARRELL

critical period for your baby's arm development has ended. **The arms are now at their proper location and proportional size for this stage in development.**

By today, you may have missed your second menstrual period.

Did You Know? The **cells in your uterus will increase** to between 17 and 40 times their nonpregnant size because they are being stimulated by extra amounts of estrogen (a hormone) and because of the stretching caused by your growing baby.

Food Facts To aid the absorption of **vitamin A,** 15 mg of **vitamin E** is recommended daily during pregnancy. Vitamin E helps prevent the breakdown of membranes that cover the blood cells and lungs and repairs damaged tissue. It also reduces the availability of LDL cholesterol, the "bad" cholesterol that forms plaque that coats the inside of the arteries and reduces bloodflow. About 60 percent of vitamin E in the diet comes directly from organic oils—safflower, corn, olive, and sunflower—and from nuts—natural almonds, sunflower seeds, hazelnuts, and peanuts. Avocado, sweet potato, olives, papaya, kale, spinach, Swiss chard, canned tomato sauce and tomato paste, and firm tofu can provide the rest.

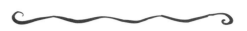

TIME TO REFLECT

Are you experiencing any pregnancy symptoms?

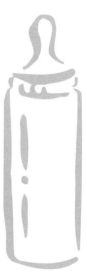

The Hebrew word for "parents" is horim, *and it comes from the same root as* moreh, *teacher. The parent is, and remains, the first and most important teacher that the child will ever have.*
RABBI KASSEL ABELSON

Week 7 Begins

DAY 43	DATE:
	223 days to go

During this week—Week 7—the cartilage that first appeared during Week 5 begins to **harden into bone** and baby's arms and legs undergo considerable change. Over the next two days, indentations will form where your baby's knees and ankles will eventually develop. The ridges on your baby's hand plates now clearly show where each finger will be. Over the next week or so, depending on the sex of your child, either testes or ovaries are forming in the pelvis. The tissue that covers the ovaries connects them to the body wall and conveys blood vessels and nerves to them. Nipples are beginning to form for both sexes. Baby's eyelids are also forming.

Varicose veins are a common side effect of pregnancy. The extra volume of blood that your body produces to support the baby as well as the extra weight you gain put pressure on the blood vessels and slow down the blood's return to the heart.

For Your Comfort **Varicose veins can be prevented or their symptoms minimized** by wearing support panty hose or leggings, elevating your legs and not crossing them when you are sitting, avoiding prolonged standing (especially while holding a baby), avoiding excessive weight gain, and by exercising (in moderation) 30 minutes a day. If you had varicose veins with your first pregnancy, you'll likely have them again.

Food Facts Because it produces a substance that is necessary for blood clotting and aids in incorporating calcium into bones, 90 mcg of **vitamin K** are recommended daily whether a woman is pregnant or not. Organic dark-green, leafy vegetables (spinach and kale), cabbage, cauliflower, broccoli, brussels sprouts, avocado, and kiwifruit are healthy natural sources of vitamin K.

For Your Information Half of the body's vitamin K is produced by bacteria in the gut; the other half is provided by foods. **Babies are routinely given a vitamin K injection at birth because they have no vitamin K–producing bacteria yet.**

DAY 44	DATE:
	222 days to go

The baby now displays another protective reflex response to touch—if an object touches the baby's head, your baby will automatically turn away. The tissues that will form the left and right sides of the brain are prominent. Semicircular canals that sense balance and body position are beginning to form in your baby's inner ear. The elbows will become visible in the next three days. By today, the indentations at your baby's knees and ankles are present. Over the next three days, the toe rays will appear.

One way to approach potential digestive discomforts is to **keep your stomach from producing extra stomach acid.** Acid indigestion is less likely if you cut out all coffee (even decaf), all carbonated beverages, all sources of caffeine (including processed chocolate ☹), all citrus fruits or juices, and dairy products.

Food Facts Pregnant women require 1,000 mg of **calcium** daily. Organic milk and organic milk products are the **richest beverage sources—** 1 cup of 2 percent milk contains 300 mg. Enriched

Life is a gift given in trust—like a child.
ANNE MORROW LINDBERGH

soy milk contains 368 mg of calcium per cup. Calcium is concentrated in cheese. One and one-half ounces (3 tablespoons) of a hard cheese like cheddar has the calcium equivalent of 1 cup of milk.

For Your Information During this week, the **baby's backbone** begins to develop the individual discs that act as cushions between each vertebra. In addition, the vertebrae in the back of the pelvis or hipbone fuse.

Did You Know? Today marks the day when the **earliest recordable brain waves** will occur.

> *What do you want to be sure to remember?*

(See page 48 for more space to write.)

DAY 45	DATE:
	221 days to go

By today or tomorrow, your baby's nipples will become visible. By now your **baby's trunk and limbs will begin to make spontaneous movements,** as the connection improves between the brain and his or her tiny muscles and nerves. You won't be able to feel any of these movements yet, because your baby is still so small, rarely comes into contact with the uterine wall, and the motions involve little actual force. Your baby now measures between ½ and ⅔ inch in length (13 to 17 mm). It might be tight, but **two babies the size of yours could play in the cap of a liter-size plastic bottle.**

Vaginal secretions respond to the hormone changes of pregnancy by becoming white and sometimes abundant. **Vaginal health** involves maintaining the balance of healthy bacteria and minimizing the growth of bacteria that contribute to vaginal, urinary tract, and yeast infections. Clean yourself a few times a day with mild soap and warm water. Never douche—douching washes away healthy bacteria. Report any changes in tissues or secretions to your health-care provider.

For Your Health Your body needs **vitamins B₆, B₁₂, folic acid, and iron to support the manufacture of red blood cells and plasma!**

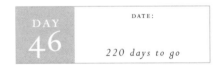

DAY 46	DATE:
	220 days to go

The cells that will form your baby's **nose develop around the nasal sacs as the facial tissues fuse to form the basic features of the face.** By today, the elbow region is clearly visible and the arms have a complete network of arteries and veins. Also by today, the toe ridges have appeared on each foot plate. The skin on the foot plate folds down between the future toes, distinguishing each from the others.

You will continue to notice breast changes: tingling sensations and tenderness. Your breasts may also feel fuller and heavier.

If there is a measure of good parenthood, it could be when your children exceed your own achievements.
TOM HAGGAI

For Your Comfort Even though sagging breasts are caused by genetics, gravity, and age, **good breast support** is crucial during pregnancy. Consider extra support provided by a nursing bra (you can use it both now and later). A professional bra fitter can help.

Food Facts About 770 mcg of **vitamin A** per day are recommended during pregnancy. All yellow, orange, and dark-green vegetables are rich in beta-carotene, a nutrient that is converted to vitamin A in the body and helps repair cell damage. The liver stores 90 percent of the body's vitamin A and keeps a 6- to 12-month supply.

DAY 47	DATE:
	219 days to go

By today, your baby's eyelids have begun to form. Over the next two days or so, your **baby's basic body proportions will change**: The trunk will begin to elongate and straighten. For the time being, most of the intestine is found in the umbilical cord since the abdominal cavity is still too small to accommodate this rapidly growing organ along with the large liver.

Are you experiencing **bloating, indigestion, and heartburn** after meals? One thing that happens during pregnancy is that the circular muscle that closes off the stomach from the esophagus relaxes and permits food and stomach acid back into the esophagus. The result is a burning sensation localized right at the end of your breastbone (in the middle of your chest) that may continue up toward your throat. If there is less food in your stomach, there is less to backwash into your esophagus.

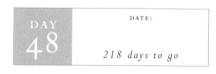

Chart your waist size and weight here and on page 181.

WAIST SIZE   WEIGHT

Did You Know? The bottom portion of your baby's stomach grows faster than the top portion, giving the stomach its characteristic curved shape.

For Your Information **Molybdenum** might be a little known trace element, but it plays an important role in helping the body use protein and sulfur. Fifty mcg is the recommended daily value during pregnancy.

Food Facts **Organic whole-grain bread, cereals, legumes, rice, grains, potatoes, and pasta** are important sources of complex carbohydrates, B vitamins, trace minerals, and fiber. One serving size equals one slice of bread, half of a bun or bagel, ½ cup cooked natural rice or other whole-grain product, or ⅔ cup ready-to-eat whole-grain cereal. Simple carbohydrates such as white bread, donuts, cookies, pretzels and chips, candy, and sweetners, have little or no nutrient value but lots of calories. They might provide a quick burst of energy, but complex carbs keep you going over time because they take longer to break down in the body.

DAY 48	DATE:
	218 days to go

The structure of your baby's **eyes** is now well developed (it's not mature enough to actually see yet, though). Over the next three days, the **tongue** will begin to develop. The external ear canal is present, and the **ears** are set low on your baby's head. As development progresses, structures

Parents learn a lot from their children about coping with life.
MURIEL SPARK

literally get pulled from one location to another. Your baby's ears will not stay low-set (unless that is a family trait). They will also migrate forward as the head grows in size and shape. Likewise, the eyes are well formed but are located on the sides of the baby's head until his face widens.

During pregnancy, **any disease you have** can be communicated to your baby, so avoid contact with people who have colds, flu, or other illnesses. As a simple precautionary step, **wash your hands whenever you transition from activities.** Natural, alcohol-free hand sanitizers do a good job, too. If a child of yours has contact with others outside the home, you're going to be exposed to a lot more germs with your second or subsequent pregnancy than during your first. Washing your child's face and hands and blocking his or her sneeze can help (the live colds and flu viruses reside in the nose).

If you think you have a cold or the flu, consult with your practitioner before you take anything for symptom relief.

Did You Know? Between 1 and 2½ teaspoons (5 to 10 ml) of amniotic fluid is now present in your uterus.

For Your Information **Even though your baby is surrounded by fluid, it does not drown** because it does not depend on its lungs for air. Oxygen comes to the baby from you through the umbilical cord blood.

DAY 49	DATE:
	217 days to go

Your baby now measures 0.62 to 0.71 inch (16 to 18 mm) long and weighs about 0.033 oz (0.94 g)—about as heavy as a U.S. dollar bill and as tall as the cap of a small tube of toothpaste! Over the next three days, your baby's arms will lengthen somewhat and begin bending at the elbow. The fingers and thumbs have appeared and are short and webbed with folds of skin in between each digit.

When women don't plan their pregnancies, it may take them about two months to notice that they haven't had a period and that something is going on. When you reflect back, you will see how much growth and change has taken place in your baby's system in these seven short weeks. **You must actively support your baby's development each and every day!**

Did You Know? The baby's arms at this point are only **as long as this printed 1!**

Food Facts **Fresh vegetables** provide vitamins, minerals, fiber, phytonutrients, and bioflavonoids and are important sources of vitamins A and C. One serving size equals 1 cup of a raw, leafy vegetable; ½ cup chopped or cooked vegetable; or ¼ cup vegetable juice.

TIME TO REFLECT
Who was the first to know you were pregnant and what were their reactions?

_____

_____

_____

_____

_____

The child supplies the power, but the parents have to do the steering.
DR. BENJAMIN SPOCK

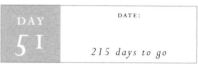

Week 8 Begins

DAY 50	DATE:
	216 days to go

DAY 51	DATE:
	215 days to go

The **surface of your baby's brain** is now beginning to develop the rounds and grooves characteristic of human brains. The **upper lip** is fully formed. Primary ossification centers that **turn cartilage into bone** are appearing in the arms and legs. This process always starts with the upper arms, where the first true bone cells appear. **If your baby is a girl**, the clitoris is beginning to form from the same tissue as the male penis.

From Week 8 on, 12 to 30 **small bumps, called Montgomery's tubercles, will appear on each areola, the colored portion of your nipple.** These tubercles are an enlargement of existing oil-bearing glands, and the oils they release help keep your nipples soft and pliable.

For Your Information The baby's heart has been beating strongly. The stomach can produce some digestive juices, the liver can manufacture blood cells, and the kidneys can extract some waste products (uric acid) from the baby's bloodstream. **Major progress is under way!**

IMPORTANT: By this time, the critical period for the baby's heart development has ended. The heart will continue to grow and develop at a slower pace.

Food Facts If you haven't already done so, **get into the habit of reading and comparing the Nutrition Facts labels on foods.** The labels provide a wealth of information, and you'll find that you're often surprised about how nutritious some foods are, while others are utterly worthless! (Nutrient comparison is a skill you'll want to pass on to your kids. After all, they may be fixing your meals when you're old!)

The retina of the eye is now fully pigmented. Your baby's arms are longer and now bend at the elbow. The fingers and thumbs have lengthened, but are still short and webbed. Notches, or grooves, have formed between the toes on the foot plate. **The baby's tail is still visible, but stubby, and disappears by the end of this week as the growth of your baby's body catches up with the early rapid growth of the spinal cord.**

You may begin to notice your clothing becoming tighter around the waist and bustline as your body changes and your baby grows. **Are you showing yet?**

Did You Know? **Attention deficit disorder, hyperactivity, learning disabilities**—each of these issues is clearly associated with children whose **mothers smoked during pregnancy** because smoking deprives babies' brains of blood and oxygen. Do you know anyone who has struggled to learn or focus or fit in? If you smoke, get the help you need to quit.

Food Facts Like vegetables, **natural fruits** provide carbohydrates, fiber, vitamins, minerals, phytonutrients, and bioflavonoids and are an important source of vitamins A and C. One serving size equals one medium piece of fruit; ½ cup chopped fruit or berries; or ¾ cup fruit juice.

IMPORTANT: Bitter melon, Rose Moss, sweet leaf, horseradish, fragrant knot weed, and pineapple are **not recommended during pregnancy** because they can bring on uterine contractions that can lead to miscarriage or early labor.

That most sensitive, most delicate of instruments: the mind of a little child.

HENRY HANDEL RICHARDSON

Childbirth Then and Now In 1652, in *The Method of Physick*, Philip Barrough recommended breathing through the pain of childbirth: "And if she was unskilled of pains of travell admonish her to hold and stop her breath strongly, and let her thrust it out to the flanks with all her might." During that time it was widely believed that birth pain could be eased if the woman would relax her pelvic region, a belief still strongly held today. (Easier said than done!)

DAY 52	DATE:
	214 days to go

By today or tomorrow, the **external ears** will be completely developed. Your baby's **nose** is stubby and the **eyes** are darkly pigmented. The bones of the **palate** are beginning to fuse and the **taste buds** are beginning to form on the surface of your baby's tongue. The **fingers have separated.** The **feet** are fan-shaped, the toes are webbed, and the **hands** touch each other as do the feet. Your baby measures 0.87 to 0.94 inch (22 to 24 mm) from crown to rump—as wide as the face of an American quarter.

The **pigmentation changes** that accompany pregnancy may become more noticeable by now. You may have noticed some blotchiness in your complexion and perhaps some darkening of the areola. These changes are temporary and will disappear once your baby is born. By this time, **the amniotic sac in your uterus is about the size of a chicken egg.**

For Your Information The appearance of the first bone cells in the baby's body marks the **end of the embryonic period.** This milestone was chosen since beginning bone formation coincides with the appearance of the basic structures and organs of the body.

Food Facts **Potassium is critical** to maintaining the heartbeat, preventing cell dehydration, and facilitating nerve cell transmission, carbohydrate metabolism, and muscle contraction. A daily dose of 4,400 mg is considered safe and adequate. A potassium supplement is usually not advised, so thankfully bananas, potatoes, figs, avocados, and blueberries are excellent natural sources.

DAY 53	DATE:
	213 days to go

At 22 to 24 mm in length, **your baby is four times as long today as it was just one month ago.** If you experienced a comparable growth rate, within a month from now you would have to duck to stand in a room with a 20-foot ceiling!

Ultrasound and MRI (magnetic resonance imaging) are the two diagnostic imaging procedures used during pregnancy because of their track record of fetal safety. X-rays are also used. If you have questions, **ask your health-care provider about the benefits and safety of these diagnostic procedures.**

Did You Know? **In boys, the development of the urinary and reproductive tracts is vitally connected.** During this eighth week, the tubes that drain urine from the boy's kidneys form a structure on each testis that help mature the sperm (epididymis) and the tube that conveys the sperm through the system (vas deferens). Ultimately, sperm and urine travel out of the body through the urethra. For girls, no such connection exists—the systems that produce ova and urine are completely separate.

For Your Health **Phosphorus** is the mineral in the second-largest quantity in the body. It combines with calcium in the bones and is part of the structure of

A sweet child is the sweetest thing in nature.

CHARLES LAMB

body cells; as you know, 700 mg is recommended daily for both pregnant and nonpregnant women. Animal protein is one of the best sources of phosphorus. **If your diet is adequate in calcium and protein, then it's adequate in phosphorus, too.**

smooth and controlled. If it's the right season, you can take your child swimming or enjoy the buoyant coolness yourself. Tai chi and yoga, with their emphasis on balance and relaxation, may be especially useful exercises during pregnancy, as is spinning on a stationary bike.

DAY 54	DATE:
	212 days to go

Your baby's **eyelids** are more developed now, and the **tongue** is fully formed. Today, the external **ears** assume their final shape, but they are still low-set. Your baby's **toes** are now unwebbed and appear longer.

The rapid rate of growth experienced by your baby during the past three to four weeks will not slow; the **pace will continue** and, at times, even quicken. **Do all you can to have the healthiest baby possible:** Be well nourished, well hydrated, well exercised, well rested, as relaxed as possible, and drug- and alcohol-free. Do what you can to reduce your exposure to pollution and contamination, and don't smoke!

For Your Information If your baby is a boy, his testes now secrete the male sex hormone (testosterone) as well as a substance to prevent his internal organs from developing into female structures. By contrast, the development of the female reproductive system does not depend on the presence of hormones or ovaries to complete its development. Either way, **development of the baby's reproductive system occurs between Weeks 8 and 12.**

Consider This Because pregnancy hormones have a tendency to soften your tendons and ligaments, you are more likely to put stress on the joints **when you exercise, so your movements should be**

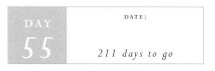

DAY 55	DATE:
	211 days to go

Over the next two days, the male **scrotum** will begin to form. The scrotum is an outpocket of the abdominal wall that houses the testes. The **head** now looks rounded and is disproportionately large, making up almost half of the baby's length. The tissue that will become the scalp has appeared as a band near the top of the baby's head. The neck region is established.

Even though your blood volume is increasing, **there will be only a slight increase in your red blood cell count.**

Did You Know? **Under the direction of the genes, the baby's development proceeds like clockwork**, with each part geared to each other part. The two ears will develop in unison, for example, in timing, and (generally) in form. However, at the same time, babies will have individually shaped ears, according to their family pattern.

Chart your waist size and weight here and on page 181.

WAIST SIZE   WEIGHT

Children think not of what is past, nor what is to come, but enjoy the present time, which few of us do.
JEAN DE LA BRUYÈRE

Food Facts Asthma and peanut, milk (lactose), and wheat gluten allergies are increasingly common among children. However, new findings suggest that women who eat about 2 tablespoons of peanut butter, 1 cup milk, 1½ slices of whole grain wheat bread, or 1¼ cups of ready-to-eat cereal or cooked wheat pasta daily during their first trimester may be able to **significantly reduce their child's tendency to develop childhood food allergies and asthma after age seven** by strengthening their immune system. Check with your practitioner about your own food sensitivities before you change your diet.

Childbirth in Other Cultures During childbirth, women of the world have pushed in the position they felt was most comfortable. Historically, in central Africa and parts of South America, women grasped a tree branch that had been fastened horizontally like a pull-up bar between two trees or two stakes driven into the ground. She hung from the bar, bent her legs at the knees into a squatting position and pushed.

DAY 56	DATE:
	210 days to go

The critical period for your baby's leg development has ended. This means that **the legs are now at their proper location** and proportional in size for this stage of development. The **shoulders** are present and have rotated out to place the arms at the sides of the body, with the elbows pointing down toward the hips. The legs have rotated in and are squarely in line with the trunk; the knees point up to the face. The **fingers and toes** are separated, and the **soles of the feet** are visible. Toe joints and toenails will be added before birth. By today, the **surface layer of the baby's skin** will begin to form. The **intestines** have begun their migration into the body cavity but are still primarily located in the umbilical cord. Your baby's external genitals are developing but don't yet look distinctly female or male. **The tail has disappeared.**

When you go to bed tonight, you will have been pregnant for two months. Right now **your uterus is about the size of a medium orange or a tennis ball.** It's amazing that so much change can take place in a baby whose movements you can't even feel yet. In another two months or so, your baby will be big enough to make his or her motions felt. Then, in addition to the symptoms of your pregnancy, you'll have a closer encounter with your growing daughter or son!

For Your Information **No longer considered an embryo, your baby is now a well-proportioned, small-scale fetus who measures about 1¹⁄₁₆ inches (27 mm) long, weighs 0.04 to 0.11 oz (1 to 3 g), and can easily be held in the bowl of a tablespoon!**

Did You Know? The baby's **umbilical cord** will grow to be about ¾ inch (19.1 mm) in diameter—about the size of an American nickel!

TIME TO REFLECT
What is the best thing about being pregnant?

_____

_____

_____

_____

The wildest colts make the best horses.
PLUTARCH

*What do you want to remember about your **Second Month**?*

Lunar Month 3

THINGS TO DO THIS MONTH:

* Eat foods from each color group—white, yellow, orange, red, green, blue, purple, even black!

* Eat whole grains and limit unhealthy fats and refined sugar.

* Consume healthy fats, which are those from olives, avocados, vegetables, and tree nuts.

* Prevent or minimize the symptoms of varicose veins.

* Avoid eating highly processed foods or those with unfamiliar, manufactured ingredients.

* Be aware of any genetic disorders in the family lines.

* Get sufficient dietary calcium.

* Avoid gaining excess weight.

* Consult with your health-care provider if you are bothered by headaches.

* Take care not to lose your balance, fall, or pass out.

* Talk to your practitioner if you have breast implants and want to breast-feed.

Week 9 Begins

DAY	DATE:
57	*209 days to go*

Over the next four days, **fingernails, toe-nails, and hair** follicles will appear (these are all specialized parts of the top layer of skin). Your baby will assume a more upright posture. The **joints** of the limbs and hips that began to develop during Week 6 now resemble adult joints.

You may find your **appetite increasing** now that some of the nausea and discomfort has stabilized. If food isn't your friend yet, look for some relief by Week 17.

Food Facts **Natural fruits and vegetables that have bright colors—yellow, orange, red, green, blue, and purple—generally contain the most phytonutrients, bioflavonoids, and nutrients.** Eat a "rainbow" variety of foods each day to maximize healthy outcomes.

Did You Know? Your baby's growth period as an embryo has just ended. From now until birth, your baby is technically called a **fetus**, from the Latin word meaning "offspring." The fetal period is a time when the baby is readied for life outside the womb—a kind of finishing period. As such, the average rate of growth until birth is 0.06 inch (1.5 mm) **per day**, with some weeks much faster than others.

DAY	DATE:
58	*208 days to go*

Your **baby's head** now makes up more than half of his or her length. For the time being, the face is broad, the eyes are widely separated, the lids are closing, and the ears are low-set. By the end of this week, your **baby will measure nearly 2 inches (5 cm) in length.** He or she stands about as high as the short side of a credit card!

As your blood volume increases, you may notice **veins becoming more visible** in your legs, breasts, and abdomen. About 20 percent of women experience varicose veins during pregnancy—veins that swell painfully because they are trying to transport so much additional blood.

For Your Comfort Try to prevent or minimize varicose veins by wearing support stockings, keeping your weight gain within the range recommended by your practitioner, elevating your feet, and exercising to improve blood flow.

Food Facts **Refined sugar is one of the most harmful "nonfoods" on the market.** It contributes nothing to the body except calories and has been linked in some way to almost every major disease, especially tooth decay, unhealthy weight gain, and diabetes. Refined sugar is found in brown sugar, white sugar, honey, maple syrup, and corn syrup. It's also found in large quantities in bakery goods, candy, soda, fruit-flavored drinks, and drinks with fruit juices like smoothies. To calculate sugar content, divide the grams of sugar in the product by 4. **The average 12 oz can of Coke or Pepsi contains 33 g or 8¼ teaspoons of sugar. *Resist!***

If you bungle raising your children, I don't think whatever else you do well matters very much.
JACQUELINE KENNEDY ONASSIS

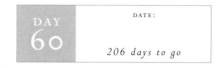

DAY 59	DATE:
	207 days to go

Your baby's body continues to straighten; his or her torso lengthens and his or her posture becomes more upright. Even though baby's legs are short and the thighs relatively small, the lower limbs are now completely webbed with blood vessels.

Your uterus is now about the size of a small grapefruit. By the end of this week, about 3 tablespoons (30 ml) of amniotic fluid bathes your baby. This fluid is renewed every three hours.

For Your Health Remember—each day you need to include 85 mg of **vitamin C** in your diet. Vitamin C helps build connective tissue for the arteries, aids in the absorption of iron, and is an antioxidant. Excellent sources of vitamin C include fresh orange juice, bell peppers, fresh grapefruit juice, brussels sprouts, broccoli, and oranges. In addition, orange juice is a good source of potassium that helps keep blood pressure at a healthy level for you and the baby.

Food Facts Fluid intake is important, but avoid **sugary soft drinks**—they contain approximately 9 teaspoons of processed sugar for every 12 oz serving. When in doubt, drink clean water.

Did You Know? All the minerals found in the ocean are the same minerals found in human blood.

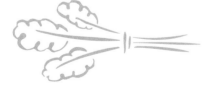

DAY 60	DATE:
	206 days to go

Over the next four days, your **baby's skin will thicken** and become less transparent. It will take another week or so for the intestines to complete their migration.

Avoid inhaling environmental **secondhand smoke from tobacco products or marijuana and exposure to other pollutants.** Smoke and pollutants enter your lungs, are carried along with the oxygen by your bloodstream, and then are transmitted to your baby's system in the oxygen–carbon dioxide exchange process. Make sure your home is well ventilated and that you operate within smoke-free environments outside your home.

IMPORTANT: Women who use **nicotine replacement devices** such as patches, inhalers, and sprays to stop smoking during pregnancy are often no more successful than women who try to quit on their own. In addition, risk to the baby is increased if she continues to smoke while using a replacement product.

For Your Information Your **calcium intake has long-term health implications** for both you and your developing baby. Calcium helps build and maintain strong bones and prevent osteoporosis, the breakdown of bony tissue. If you're at least 30 years old or will be soon, bone loss may have already started if you smoke or are around smokers, use alcohol to excess or binge, have a diet low in calcium, or get inadequate physical exercise.

You have to love your children unselfishly. That's hard, but it's the only way.
BARBARA BUSH

DAY 61	DATE: *205 days to go*

The colored portion of the eye (the **iris**) will begin to develop over the next three days. Over the next two days, the **eyelids** will meet and temporarily fuse shut.

Consistent with **pigmentation changes** during pregnancy, you may notice that your moles, freckles, recent scars, or dark birthmarks are darkening along with your cervix and vulva. This is quite predictable and temporary.

If you are age 35 or older or at high risk for genetic disorders, your health-care provider may recommend that some **diagnostic screening tests** be done in the next 10 weeks or so. Be sure to ask questions, express any concerns, and gather enough information to evaluate the risks and benefits of these procedures for you and your baby.

Consider This **The darkening of the nipples in preparation for breast-feeding may make it easier for the baby to spot the food source.**

Childbirth in Other Cultures The tradition in southern Africa is for women to squat during labor, knees wide apart, ankles together, with heels supporting the area between the vagina and anus to prevent tearing.

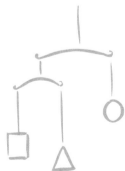

DAY 62	DATE: *204 days to go*

Ossification centers are established in the **skull**; those in the long bones continue to develop as your baby becomes more solid. Your baby's **bones and muscles are growing rapidly**, and his or her developing body begins to attain proportions more like a newborn's.

Although **weight gain** fluctuates from week to week, your average weight gain is about 1 lb a week (⅔ lb weekly if you were overweight when you got pregnant).

Food Facts **To support the baby's production of cartilage and bone tissue**, three to four servings of calcium-containing foods will probably satisfy the 1,000 mg daily requirement. In addition to fortified milk and yogurt, other excellent food sources of calcium include cheese (especially Swiss, provolone, and Monterey Jack), wild salmon, and broccoli.

Consider This The calcium and protein found in low-fat milk, along with regular exercise, **might help with weight loss after the baby is born. Better yet, you'll burn 500 kcal per day sitting down and breast-feeding your baby!**

Childbirth in Other Cultures In northern Russia during the 1800s, it was customary for the midwife to require the laboring woman and her husband to name the people, beside their spouse, with whom they had slept. If the labor was easy, all had told the truth; if labor was difficult, one of them had lied about an affair.

The illusions of childhood are necessary experiences: a child should not be denied a balloon because an adult knows that sooner or later it will burst.

MARCELENE COX

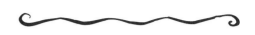

DAY 63

DATE:

203 days to go

The skin has become thicker and less transparent. The **vagina** is beginning to develop in females. The **penis** is now distinguishable in males. Your baby has now attained a more upright posture. In one short week, your **baby more than doubled his or her weight**, to between ¼ and ⅓ oz (7.6 g).

Every baby shows distinct individuality in behavior. This is because the actual structure of the muscles varies slightly from baby to baby. The alignment of the muscles in the face, for example, follows an inherited pattern. **The facial expressions of the baby are already similar to the facial expressions of the parents.**

Food Facts **Sodium** is an element found in table salt. Along with potassium, sodium permits nerve cell transmission and muscle contraction. The **highest concentration** is in foods such as pickles, potato chips and other snacks, hot dogs, and deli meats, wherein sodium is used as a preservative.

Childbirth Then and Now The first attempt to make newborn feedings follow a schedule was based on Dr. T. S. Southworth's observations in 1906. He recommended ten nursings a day for the first month and eight a day in the second and third months. Today, nursing more frequently (8 to 18 feedings per day in the first weeks) improves milk production and reduces nipple soreness.

Chart your waist size and weight here and on page 181.

WAIST SIZE   WEIGHT

TIME TO REFLECT

What has changed the most since you've been pregnant?

What do you want to be sure to remember?

(See page 66 for more space to write.)

God could not be everywhere, and therefore he created mothers.

JEWISH PROVERB

DAY 64	DATE:
	202 days to go

Sometime during the next three weeks, the urine that is formed by your **baby's kidneys** will be excreted into the amniotic fluid. The urine is sterile and is carried away in the regular replacement of the fluid. By late pregnancy, about a half liter (a little over 2¼ cups) of urine is added daily!

You have probably **gained 2 to 4 lb (1–1.8 kilos)** by now. If you were underweight when you began your pregnancy, you will gain a little more than other women; overweight women will gain a little less. Women tend to gain more with a second or subsequent baby than with their first and may carry that weight differently.

To an extent, recommendations regarding weight gain are based on a woman's BMI (body mass index) when she began her pregnancy. Forty pounds is considered an upper limit on healthy weight gain for women who began their pregnancies in good health and had BMIs under 30. Women who are over or under healthy BMI ranges should be individually assessed. No matter where you fall on the BMI spectrum, **report any sudden, large weight gain to your practitioner**, since it might be tied to fluid retention and changes in your blood pressure.

For Your Health Almost all the non-fluid weight gained during a healthy pregnancy is lean tissue: placenta, uterus, milk-producing glands, and, of course, the baby. **Excess weight affects both of you.** For your baby, unhealthy weight gain is associated with a tendency toward later obesity, breathing problems, unstable blood-sugar levels, and unhealthy high blood pressure. For you, too much weight gained is associated with the risk of unsafe blood pressure changes,
gestational diabetes, additional back and leg pain, damage to the birth canal (vagina), and a baby too big for vaginal delivery.

Food Facts Women who get their fats mostly from olives, vegetables, and tree nuts lose more weight after childbirth and keep it off longer than women on low-fat diets. That finding makes sense because **the Nutrition Facts labels on low- or fat-free foods reveal calories in the form of carbohydrates and sugars.** For example, 1 cup (240 ml) of low-fat ice cream still has 250 to 350 calories. **It takes only 3,400 extra calories to gain a pound of weight.**

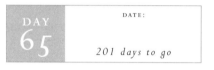

DAY 65	DATE:
	201 days to go

Over the next three days, your baby's **fingernails** will begin to grow from the nail beds. The **baby's skin is sensitive all over**—any type of touch causes your baby to move.

About 90 percent of all women will develop **stretch marks** at some time during their pregnancy. If you have elastic, well-toned skin and try to keep weight gain steady and gradual, your chance of developing stretch marks will be reduced.

Did You Know? Good skin tone, good nutrition, hydration to encourage **skin elasticity**, and gradual (not rapid and not excessive) weight gain can prevent or minimize stretch marks. If you got stretch marks the first time, you probably won't get more with subsequent pregnancies unless you gain significantly more weight or carry your weight in a different area.

Don't be discouraged if your children reject your advice. Years later they will offer it to their own offspring.

OSCAR WILDE

Food Facts **Sulfur** is in every cell in your body. Your body's most rigid protein—your skin, hair, nails, joint pads, and cartilage in your nose—has a high sulfur content. Currently, there is no recommended daily intake for sulfur, and sulfur deficiencies are generally unknown. The primary animal source of sulfur is egg yolk. One caution: **check with your practitioner before you use sulfur-based acne treatments on your skin.**

What do you want to be sure to remember?

(See page 66 for more space to write.)

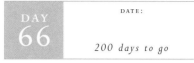

DAY 66	DATE:
	200 days to go

Your baby's brain now has the same structure it will have at birth; it's just a smaller size. Between now and Week 16, the mechanism that enables the baby's sense of smell (the olfactory system) is developing. The thyroid, pancreas, and gall bladder will complete their development during the next three days.

With rare exceptions, you won't feel your lively baby move yet. The baby's newly formed muscles are weak, and your baby is so small that the womb has barely expanded and is still contained within the framework of your hips.

Food Facts Foods of animal origin, such as meat, poultry, fish, eggs, cheese, and milk, are excellent sources of B vitamins and provide complete **protein.** Legumes (dried beans, peas, and lentils), nuts, and seeds must be eaten in combination with whole grains in order to obtain the essential building blocks of protein in their proper balance. Ground turkey makes the leanest ground meat; chopped sirloin makes the leanest ground beef, followed by ground chuck. To avoid illness associated with **undercooked ground meat**, make sure it is well done.

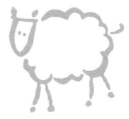

In the all-important world of family relations, three words are almost as powerful as the famous "I love you." They are "Maybe you're right."

OREN ARNOLD

DAY **67**

DATE:

199 days to go

A new reflex is present: Now when your baby's face is touched, he or she will open his or her mouth. This is called the **rooting reflex** and helps babies find the food source. The tooth buds for the **permanent teeth** begin to form this week, as do the membranes that will become the **vocal cords.**

You may notice an occasional **headache.** Headaches during pregnancy are generally caused by hormonal changes, added stress, and increased sinus congestion. Talk to your health-care provider about your headaches if they start to interfere with what you need to do.

IMPORTANT: Don't take any medication without your practitioner's approval.

Childbirth in Other Cultures Historically, women living in Mexico's Yucatán Peninsula gave birth in the matrimonial hammock, the traditional bed of the couples of the region. The midwife was positioned on a low stool in front of the hammock.

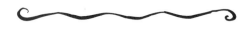

TIME TO REFLECT
What have you noticed about your appetite?

DAY **68**

DATE:

198 days to go

Your baby's thyroid, pancreas, and gall bladder have now completed their development. Within the next three days, the hard, bony part of the palate is completely formed and the pancreas begins to secrete insulin.

As **your blood pressure decreases** because pregnancy hormones relax the walls of the blood vessels, **you may feel light-headed and dizzy.** Change positions slowly, especially if you are getting up from lying down. Make sure you're stable before you stand. If you feel unstable on your feet, sit down or lie down as soon as you can. Elevate your feet (ideally, higher than your heart). Take your time. The obvious goal is to keep you from passing out and falling down. Your baby's pretty well protected, but you could bump your head and hurt yourself.

 If you faint, contact your practitioner. They'll want to know more about the cause.

Childbirth in Other Cultures Some tribal societies in New Guinea have different ideas about how long a pregnancy should last. They believe that a child could be born anytime the child decided to be, which can sometimes lead to confusion. If a man has been away from home for a year and a baby is born to his wife three months after his return, he may not question her fidelity. He may believe the baby hurried up to see its father's face!

Chart your waist size and weight here and on page 181.

WAIST SIZE   WEIGHT

Wouldn't it be wonderful to be as brilliant as our children thought we were when they were young, and only half as stupid as they think we are when they're teenagers?
DAISY BROWN

DAY 69	DATE:
	197 days to go

Over the next two days, the muscles in the walls of your **baby's digestive tract** will become functional in order to begin practicing the movements required to **push food** from one portion of the body to another. Some intestinal coils may remain in the umbilical cord, but most are repositioned in the abdomen.

Despite occasional light-headedness, **you may feel more emotionally stable now** as your body gets more and more used to being pregnant. Every woman is different, however, and each pregnancy is unique, no matter how many children you have had.

Food Facts Iron is an important element in pregnancy. **Vitamin C and copper** facilitate the absorption of iron from foods. The **recycling of iron** from old red blood cells is quite efficient, with 90 percent of the iron being reused in the synthesis of new red blood cells. Copper is available from almost all foods, and vitamin C is abundant in fresh citrus. As you know, cooking with unglazed cast-iron cookware may provide additional iron.

Childbirth Then and Now The Greek physician Hippocrates devised a test he believed would reveal the sex of a developing child: If the woman's right breast was firmer or her right eye was brighter, she would have a boy; if her left breast was firmer or the left eye brighter, she would have a girl. Another conviction was that boys sat higher in the womb than girls, an unfounded belief that lasted well into the twentieth century.

DAY 70	DATE:
	196 days to go

The hard, bony part of baby's palate is now completely formed. This bony plate divides the mouth from the nose and makes it possible to eat and breathe at the same time. Your **baby's growth rate has slowed somewhat**. His or her weight has doubled in the last week to almost ½ oz (14 g); its length has increased to about 2½ inches (63 mm).

Most **breast implants involve a soft silicone- or saltwater-filled pouch.** Breast implants should not affect a woman's ability to breast-feed, but may reduce milk production. The mammary gland itself is not disturbed, especially if the implant is situated under the chest muscles. The best incision sites for successful breast-feeding are under the breast or in the armpit. However, the safety of silicone-filled implants is still uncertain. Implants filled with silicone may be reactive and place the mother and/or her baby at risk for exposure to toxic substances when they leak. **A woman's best source of information on breast implants is her health-care provider.**

Consider This If you are considering breast augmentation, the **most cautious approach** may be to wait until you're finished having children. At that point, gather as much information as you possibly can before you decide.

Food Facts Diluted, pure 100 percent **apple juice** is an excellent beverage to drink during pregnancy. Natural apple juice is a good source of iron, potassium, and magnesium. Consider diluting it with water. Better yet, eat a fresh, raw apple. It provides fiber to aid digestion and all the nutrient value of unprocessed food with 40 percent less sugar and calories than juice.

Small children disturb your sleep, big children your life.
YIDDISH PROVERB

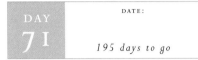
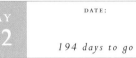

DAY 7 1	DATE:
	195 days to go

DAY 7 2	DATE:
	194 days to go

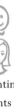

Sometime during the next two weeks, the urine that is formed by your baby's kidneys will be excreted into the amniotic fluid. Each kidney contains about 800,000 delicate *nephrons*, or waste-screening cells.

Select **comfortable clothes** that don't restrict your movement or inadvertently cut off your circulation or bind you at the waist. There are lots of fashion-forward looks in sustainable maternity wear, if that's your interest. No matter what you choose, wear something you feel comfortable in.

Childbirth Then and Now In England from 1705 on, women were urged to have a healthy pregnancy by moderating their diets, sleeping as much as possible, and not wearing tight corsets. Cordials containing cinnamon, nutmeg, sugar, and eggs were served to warm and strengthen the mother-to-be.

Food Facts **Dried fruits** are a concentrated form of the sugars, calories, and nutrients found in fresh fruit. For example, ¼ cup of raisins contains 124 calories, tons of fiber and iron, but also the equivalent of more than 7 teaspoons (29 grams) of sugar! (Craisins are similar, but start out as cranberries, not grapes.) When you're hungry for candy, eat dried fruit instead—at least it started out fresh!

All of your baby's intestines have now migrated in the abdomen.

Just as in the past two months, **you will continue to feel more tired than usual.** Continue to listen to your body and make adjustments in your schedule so you can rest when you need to.

For Your Information Stay away from **dried bananas** since they're processed in oil and loaded with fat.

Food Facts Bell peppers are an excellent source of vitamin C. Depending on what color and flavor is desired, bell peppers are harvested at different stages to produce green, red, and orange bell peppers. **Green bells have two times the amount of vitamin C by weight as citrus fruits; red bells have three times the vitamin C and are also a good source of vitamin A.**

What do you want to be sure to remember?

(See page 66 for more space to write.)

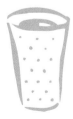

If there must be trouble, let it be in my day, that my child may have peace.

THOMAS PAINE

58

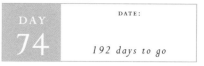

DAY 73	DATE:
	193 days to go

The **placenta** grows with the baby, but not as fast. At this point in development, it weighs around 1 oz (28 g); at the time of birth, it will weigh between 1 and 2 lb (448 to 896 g).

If you are experiencing food aversions and just can't stomach certain foods or food groups, **make sure you're not suffering any nutrient, vitamin, or mineral losses as a consequence.**

Childbirth in Other Cultures For Australian aborigines, childbirth is women's business. When a woman is ready to give birth, she leaves her home camp and her female elders take her to a special place. Giving birth on the land is considered a spiritual experience that creates a bond among the mother, her child, and the earth.

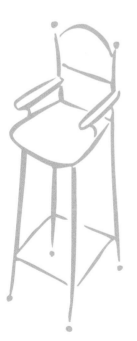

DAY 74	DATE:
	192 days to go

Over the next three days, the vocal cords will form in your baby's *larynx*, or voice box. **The baby will not be able to make sounds**, however, or cry out loud until the amniotic fluid is replaced by air after birth.

Pregnancy makes women more prone to **bladder infections**, and the longer urine stays in the bladder, the more likely it is to grow bacteria if such bacteria are present. Drink plenty of fluids to flush out your system—purified water is best. Don't hold your urine, and when you do go, empty your bladder completely. For better hygiene, wash your hands before and after you urinate or have sex, and wipe from front to back with a baby wipe. (Dispose of wipes responsibly.) Always urinate after sex to help cleanse the urethra.

For Your Health **These signs need to be reported to your health-care provider,** as they might indicate a bladder infection: pain and burning during urination, urgency or needing to pee frequently, blood in the urine, or a strong odor.

IMPORTANT: An **untreated bladder infection won't just go away.** Instead, the kidneys might become infected, and damage to their delicate screening structures is a serious consequence. **Don't wait to report any symptoms.**

If we could learn how to utilize all the intelligence and patent goodwill children are born with, instead of ignoring much of it—why—there might be enough to go around!
DOROTHY CANFIELD FISHER

DAY	DATE:
75	*191 days to go*

By today, all of your baby's **20 baby teeth** and their sockets have formed in the gums. Over the next three days, the **intestines** will form into folds and become lined with *villi* (small, finger-like projections in the lining of the intestines that absorb certain nutrients).

Very hot baths or showers during pregnancy may be exhausting and may cause fainting. Spas and hot tubs should be avoided if the temperature is higher than 100°F (38°C).

Food Facts Vitamin C is not stored in the body's tissues and continually has to be resupplied. Fifty percent of **vitamin C is destroyed** by cooking and processing, so eat raw fruits and vegetables and drink fresh juices.

Childbirth in Other Cultures Among the Arapesh of Papua New Guinea, fresh coconuts are reserved for tribal feasts and for women who are breast-feeding.

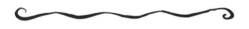

DAY	DATE:
76	*190 days to go*

By today, your baby's **vocal cords** will have formed in the larynx. In another week, the primary ossification centers will appear in the middle of nearly all the **bones of the limbs.** Ossification sites also develop in the bones of the knee and in the ends of the thigh bones and the bones of the lower leg.

A woman's **carbohydrate** intake (including sugars, starches, and fiber) is usually more than adequate during pregnancy.

Food Facts **Legumes** (which include dried beans, peas, and lentils) are one of the best food values during pregnancy. They offer high-quality protein that is rich in iron, thiamin (B_1), and riboflavin (B_2). One cup of prepared dried beans or peas provides 15 to 20 mg of protein, about one-fourth of the 71 g of protein required daily during pregnancy.

Did You Know? The growth needs of the newborn baby are *exactly met* by the protein mixture in the mother's milk.

TIME TO REFLECT
What have you noticed about your sleep patterns?

And do respect the women of the world; remember you all had mothers.
ALLEN TOUSSAINT

| DAY 77 | DATE:
189 days to go |

By this time, your **baby's liver** will have begun to secrete bile and the pancreas will have begun to produce insulin. The **intestines** have formed into folds and are lined with nutrient-extracting villi. Bile is produced by the liver but is stored in a small sac called the **gall bladder** (already formed). (When there is food in the small intestine, the bile will be released into the intestine to help digest fatty foods.)

By this time, you may have experienced some **back pain**—it often begins before Week 12 of pregnancy. The chief cause is the production of relaxin, a hormone that allows your pelvis to expand to accommodate the growing uterus and encourages the joints connecting the hips to the backbone to loosen to make childbirth easier. Relaxin production peaks at Week 14 and remains fairly high until 48 hours after birth.

For Your Information Back pain is common during pregnancy. Women who have scoliosis, who had back pain prior to pregnancy, or who already have a toddler are most likely to experience severe discomfort.

Did You Know? Although bone appears solid and motionless, it is active, living tissue. Around 700 mg of calcium is renewed in the bone tissue each day, so a fresh supply needs to be constantly available. **Remember, the recommended daily value for calcium during pregnancy is 1,000 mg.**

Chart your waist size and weight here and on page 181.

WAIST SIZE   WEIGHT

What do you want to be sure to remember?

(See page 66 for more space to write.)

What war is to man, childbirth is to woman.

HINDU PROVERB

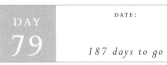

DAY 78	DATE:
	188 days to go

Your **baby's hand** is becoming more and more functional. The baby is beginning to move his or her thumb in opposition to the other fingers. Over the next three days, the **external sex structures** of girl babies can be clearly distinguished from those of boys. During this week, in-growth of the head of the penis occurs. When that in-growth stops, the **foreskin**, a double-thickness sleeve of skin covering the penis, has formed.

Once a woman becomes physically and emotionally adjusted to the impact of pregnancy, she generally enjoys **a feeling of well-being**—her appetite is good, and she looks and feels well. This well-being can only be experienced, however, if you are healthy, well nourished, relaxed, and not overly tired.

Childbirth Then and Now Many early agricultural societies believed that life was created when the sky or heaven (which was considered to be male) showered rain on the earth (considered to be female).

Did You Know? An **e-cigarette or vape pen** uses a battery to turn nicotine and other chemicals into a vapor, which is then inhaled. These devices still deliver nicotine to unborn babies like conventional cigarettes do, along with unknown types and amounts of other chemicals. **Vaping is NOT safe during pregnancy.**

DAY 79	DATE:
	187 days to go

In the womb, your baby **practices inhaling and exhaling** movements that send amniotic fluid in and out of its lungs. The presence of the fluid is essential to the proper formation of the air sacs within the lungs.

By this time, you will probably have noticed some **darkening** of the area around the nipple (called the areola) and some enlargement of its diameter. And, if this is your **second pregnancy**, you may be starting to show already. Your uterus is likely to expand out of your pelvis sooner the second time, so you may not experience as much frequent urination. But, you may be showing earlier and wearing maternity clothes before the 12th week since your muscles have been stretched by the first pregnancy, even though exercise may have regained the shape of your abdomen.

For Your Information The burning sensation called "heartburn" has nothing to do with your heart.

Childbirth in Other Cultures In societies where men have never been allowed to witness childbirth, men fantasize about the terrible nature of birth. Traditionally, the Arapesh men of Papua New Guinea give pantomimed accounts of childbirth where women are depicted as writhing around in screaming agony. In reality, the Arapesh women give birth quietly and matter-of-factly on the damp ground of a steep slope in the dark with no one to help them but one other young woman. The new mother is expected to care for the newborn all by herself.

Food Facts The **larger portions** served in some restaurants can be turned into multiple, smaller meals

Never try to make your son or daughter another you; one is enough!
ARNOLD GLASOW

by asking for a take-home container as soon as you get your food and cutting portions in half. Eat half and take home the rest for later. Smaller meals every two hours help maintain a steady flow of nutrients.

DAY 80	DATE:
	186 days to go

The baby's **large intestine** (colon) rotates 180 degrees counterclockwise and forms a square around the small intestine, much like a frame surrounds a picture. The two top corners of the colon attach to the body wall and with the anus, while the small intestine remains suspended in the abdomen.

You may continue to notice some **discomfort after eating.** Think about cutting out foods that provoke indigestion—like spicy, greasy, or fatty foods, tomato products, citrus juice, peppermint, spearmint, onion, and garlic—or eat smaller portions. These foods relax the muscle that closes the stomach off from your throat, causing burning, bloating, and the feeling of food coming back up from the stomach. Chances are you can go back to eating these foods after the baby is born.

IMPORTANT: Remember that your baby is hungry even though you might not be. Eat small meals every two hours rather than skipping meals or eating only a couple large portions.

For Your Information In addition to back and pelvic pain, relaxin can also cause changes in the nerve that runs through the area of **your wrist** called the carpal tunnel. Symptoms include tingling, numbness, and/or pain in the thumb, index, and middle finger; and a sensation of weakness when you button, zip, or try to lift something with your wrist, like your

water glass or a pot on the stove. Like diabetes, carpal tunnel syndrome can be brought on by pregnancy. Report these symptoms to your practitioner for evaluation.

Food Facts The **healthy balance of beneficial bacteria** in the digestive tract can be disturbed by diets high in meat-derived protein, sugars, and sweets, and low in dairy foods, dietary fiber, and vegetables and fruits. The resulting imbalance and growth of less healthy microorganisms can produce diarrhea and gastrointestinal upset and contribute to the development of food allergies. Foods like probiotics in natural yogurt can do a lot to restore balance to the digestive tract. Be sure to check the levels of active live cultures in your yogurt—the more live cultures there are, the more you stand to benefit.

TIME TO REFLECT
Have you had any dreams about your baby?

_____

_____

_____

_____

DAY 81	DATE:
	185 days to go

Over the next three days, your **baby's spleen** will assume functions supervised by the liver: the removal of old red blood cells and the production of antibodies.

Parents are like shuttles on a loom. They join the threads of the past with the threads of the future and weave their own bright patterns as they go.

FRED ROGERS

You may notice some **constipation.** As the pregnancy hormones relax the muscles of your bowel, moving solid waste through your system is made slower and less efficient. Also, your growing uterus presses on the bowel and further interferes with its activity.

For Your Health **What to do about constipation?** Exercise gets your body and bowel moving. Engage in physical activity that's easy on your joints, such as walking or swimming, and respond promptly to the urge to poop. Eating prunes, prune juice, and figs may also be helpful, as are warm or hot fluids right after getting up.

Food Facts **When heart problems occur, magnesium is the most likely nutrient to be missing from the person's diet.**

DAY 82	DATE:
	184 days to go

Much progress has taken place in the development of your **baby's mouth.** The bony palate, or roof of the mouth, has been complete for some weeks, the sucking muscles are filling out the cheeks, the tooth buds are under the gums, and the esophagus, windpipe, and larynx are present. By today, the baby's salivary glands will begin to function. Over the next three days, your baby will begin to make breathing, sucking, and swallowing motions!

By this time, most pregnant women can see a clear **pattern of dilated veins** on their chest and breasts.

Food Facts **Unprocessed raw cacao beans (from which all chocolate is made) and raw cocoa powder** are good sources of vitamin C, manganese, magnesium, potassium, iron, chromium, and zinc. It is naturally sugar-free, and its fat contains omega-6 fatty acids. Some researchers contend that raw chocolate contains a stimulant substance (theobromine), but that caffeine does not occur naturally in chocolate products.

Childbirth in Other Cultures When Maori women of New Zealand give birth, they traditionally deliver on the ground near a stream. The Maori word *whenna* means both "earth" and "placenta."

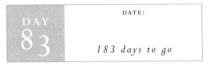

DAY 83	DATE:
	183 days to go

Baby's **arms** have almost reached their final proportions relative to body size, but baby's **legs** are still quite short. In fact, the arms and legs are about the same length. The **spleen** is now fully functional.

You've probably seen your practitioner two or three times by now. Soon, prenatal visits will become a predictable part of your routine. **Make sure you write down questions you want to ask as well as symptoms you are experiencing so your practitioner can answer your questions and evaluate any changes.**

IMPORTANT: Adding **extra fiber** to your diet and **foods that contain a lot of water** are other natural remedies for constipation. Select foods like watermelon, oranges, cucumbers, and celery. Check with your practitioner before taking any over-the-counter preparations.

For Your Information During your pregnancy, your uterus will increase in weight from approximately 1 oz (28 g) to more than 2¼ lb (1.13 kg)—**more than 360 times its original weight!**

Children are natural mimics—they act like their parents in spite of every attempt to teach them good manners.
ANONYMOUS

Food Facts **Zinc is a trace element of critical importance during pregnancy.** It forms part of the structure of bone and is involved in DNA and protein production, immune reactions, breaking down blood sugar into usable energy, the utilization of vitamin A, wound healing, and protecting the development of the brain and nervous system. The recommended daily value of zinc during pregnancy is 11 mg and should vary little from that amount. The ingestion of too much zinc (over time, not just during pregnancy) can limit immune protection and block the absorption of copper. The ingestion of too much **folic acid** during pregnancy, however, can block the absorption of zinc. Limiting daily folic acid intake to no more than 800 mg with zinc at 11 mg should balance the equation. Check with your health-care provider if you have concerns.

> *Chart your waist size and weight here and on page 181.*

WAIST SIZE   WEIGHT

DATE:

DAY 84

182 days to go

Your **baby is now quite active** and his or her muscle responses are less mechanical and puppetlike and more smooth and fluid, like a newborn's. Do you remember that at the end of the second month, the baby measured about l inch (27 mm) in length and weighed about as much as a U.S. dollar bill (1g or 0.04 oz)? Now, he or she is 3 times as long and more than 50 times as heavy! Hmm. Fifty bucks worth of weight!

This day marks the end of the third full month of pregnancy—**one full trimester**, one third of your baby's total gestational time. **Each day that you read, reflect, think, and learn about your pregnancy and your unborn child, you come closer to understanding how to supply the needs of your developing baby and to assimilating into the role of new (or renewed) parent.**

Food Facts The amount of magnesium that can be found in the body of a 130-lb person is only about 1¾ oz (50 g), and most of that is in the bones. This observation might lead you to believe that magnesium is a minor nutrient, but think again. **Magnesium and potassium** are critical at the level of the cell: Magnesium helps build and repair tissue while potassium maintains the fluid and chemical balance in cells. By itself, magnesium builds bones and teeth, helps control cholesterol levels, and balances blood-sugar levels. Magnesium keeps the uterine muscles from contracting prematurely and helps regularize the heartbeat. The recommended daily value of magnesium during pregnancy is 360 mg.

Did You Know? **The accuracy of your estimated due date can be confirmed by examining the size of your uterus** during prenatal visits. If there seems to be a large difference between the actual size and the expected size of the uterus, **an ultrasound picture may be used to measure the width of your baby's head and thighbone.**

Young children and chickens would ever be eating.
THOMAS TUSSER

Lunar Month 4

THINGS TO DO THIS MONTH:

* Sleep or rest on your left side to improve circulation.

* Consider including (more) soy-based and fresh foods in your diet.

* Eat tree nuts every other day (just not daily).

* Report any hand, foot, face, or ankle swelling to your health-care provider.

* Reduce nasal congestion; check any over-the-counter meds with your practitioner.

* Avoid eating liver when you're pregnant.

* No caffeine, alcohol, smoking/vaping/marijuana, or unprescribed drugs.

* Eat organic foods whenever possible.

* Exercise, even if it's just walking and stretching.

* Drink lots of clean, fresh water.

* If you want something really sweet, eat dried fruit.

* Carry a snack with you so your blood-sugar level doesn't drop too low.

* If you're pregnant during cold and flu season, ask about preventive measures.

* Don't exceed the recommended daily allowance for vitamin A, but take your prenatal vitamins faithfully.

* Consider non-diagnostic 3-D/4-D ultrasound portraiture.

Week 13 Begins

DAY 85	DATE: *181 days to go*

Your **baby's neck** is now well defined. The head now rests on the neck instead of the shoulders.

Your baby needs you to eat sufficient, well-balanced healthy meals and snacks and to drink plenty of fluids. In addition, your growing uterus is getting big enough to press on a major blood vessel to the right of your spine (the vena cava) when you lie on your back. **To maintain optimal circulation, try to sleep or rest on your left side.**

Did You Know? You should know that nothing your practitioner does affects the cosmetic appearance of your **baby's belly button** or whether it points in or out. The strength of the baby's tissues at the umbilical site determines this at birth.

Childbirth in Other Cultures Canadian Eskimos traditionally believe that the spirit or life force enters a baby early in the pregnancy and that the mother can talk to it and teach it during that time.

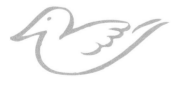

DAY 86	DATE: *180 days to go*

Over the next three days, the **baby's scalp hair pattern** will be determined. Your baby is now able to practice breathing, swallowing, and sucking movements in **preparation for life outside the womb.** Some amniotic fluid is swallowed and processed by your baby's maturing digestive tract, practicing for the time when he or she will drink milk.

Along with your efforts, your body naturally works to reduce the risks associated with pregnancy by increasing blood volume, increasing red blood cell count, getting more oxygen to tissues, and improving blood-clotting ability.

For Your Information As **marijuana use** becomes more common, its impact on the baby's development before birth becomes more important. Babies born to mothers who smoked marijuana during pregnancy are more likely to develop **learning, attention, and memory problems** than babies born to non-smokers. These findings suggest that the baby's brain and nervous system are affected by marijuana's active ingredients and other known and unknown plant-related chemicals and substances used in processing. **There is currently *no* safe level of marijuana use during pregnancy.**

Childbirth in Other Cultures According to Mayan tradition, a woman who gives birth sleeps with her newborn in her arms and will not be separated from the baby until the mother resumes normal activities 20 days later.

If any of us had a child that we thought was as bad as we know we were, we would have cause to start to worry.
WILL ROGERS

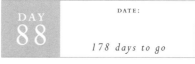

DAY 87

DATE:

179 days to go

The rapid and sustained growth experienced by the baby this month enables him or her to be **more agile** than before. For example, your baby can now turn his or her head, open his or her mouth, and press his or her lips together. Not bad for somebody who only weighs about as much as a slice of whole wheat bread (1 oz or 28 g) and stands only 3⅜ inches (8.5 cm) tall!

During pregnancy, your organ systems receive additional blood, according to their increased workload. Blood flow to the uterus and kidneys is increased, while blood flow to the liver and brain remains the same.

IMPORTANT: You'll want to continue with your program of regular, moderate exercise, but avoid cycling, skiing, roller-blading, horseback riding, skateboarding, and surfing, because even experienced athletes can fall. Even though your baby is well protected, you'll want to **avoid jarring your uterus.** In addition, intense physical activity can reduce blood flow to the placenta.

Food Facts **Soy is the main source of phosphatidylserine which keeps nerve cell membranes from breaking down.** As such, it may reduce the risk of Alzheimer's disease and help with learning and memory. Foods containing at least 6.25 g of soy protein per serving may make a significant difference. Ask your health-care provider about the potential benefits of soy foods for you and your baby.

Chart your waist size and weight here and on page 181.

WAIST SIZE   WEIGHT

DAY 88

DATE:

178 days to go

By today, your baby's scalp hair pattern has been determined.

You should feel less breast tenderness and tingling this month. **Women generally feel more comfortable during the second trimester** (Months 4, 5, and 6).

Food Facts **Oatmeal has superfood properties.** One cup of natural rolled-oat oatmeal provides a significant amount of protein (5 g), 1.4 mg of iron, and half of the vitamin B_1 you require each day during pregnancy, plus protection for your heart, fiber to help control blood sugar levels and protect your bowel, antioxidant protection, and help with weight control. The instant flavored varieties have lots of sugar and other additives you don't need. Add your own fresh fruit, like blueberries, and your own flavoring, like ground cinnamon, and make your oatmeal even more nutritious.

Childbirth Then and Now Starting in the eighteenth century, Western women were advised by their physicians to restrict food intake during pregnancy in order to keep from gaining too much weight. At that time, malnutrition was prevalent, and malnourished girls often developed narrow, misshapen pelvises. Since such a pelvis made it difficult if not impossible to deliver a normal-size baby and threatened the life of both the mother and the child, all women (even well-nourished ones) were encouraged to limit protein, calorie, salt, and carbohydrate intake during pregnancy. We know now that women should not diet during pregnancy, but such advice was widespread in the United States even as late as the 1960s.

Listen to little children carefully and you will learn great things.

G. WEINBERG

DAY 89	DATE:
	177 days to go

Your baby now displays **some impressive hand and arm movements**, such as making a fist, moving the thumbs, bending the wrists, and grasping. All the body movements that the baby engages in right now constitute practice. It takes some time for the nervous system and the muscles to make smooth, synchronous movements. So these motions test the hookups within the neuromuscular system. Your baby also is exercising his or her tiny muscles by moving them.

By now you may be experiencing **some mild swelling** or edema. It will be most noticeable in your ankles and feet, because of the effect of gravity on your tissues.

Swelling is an important symptom to report to your health-care provider during your checkup or by phone. Keep a record of swelling that occurs in the ankles, feet, hands, or face.

Childbirth in Other Cultures In the villages of Jordan in the Middle East, inhabitants advise that people be as careful of the child within its mother's womb as they are of the chicken in the egg.

For Your Comfort **Elevate your feet** when you sit and avoid standing for prolonged periods of time. **Stay well hydrated** and **exercise** to keep fluid circulating.

DAY 90	DATE:
	176 days to go

Your baby's **heart pumps** about 6 gallons or 25 qt of blood a day during the fourth month; that rate will increase to 300 qt of blood a day by the time he or she is born—enough to fill a large rain barrel.

By the end of this month, **your growing uterus** will rise out of the confines of your hipbones. Even though your baby is moving quite a bit, you still can't feel the movements because the baby doesn't bump into the walls of your uterus and doesn't have much muscle strength. While these movements are visible during ultrasound examination, you'll first detect the baby's movements in another seven weeks or so. It's ironic that while most mothers really want to feel their baby move and are so pleased when they finally do, those same movements will eventually keep them up at night and bump so hard they'd think their baby is wearing boots!

Childbirth in Other Cultures The Bambara of Africa and other African tribal groups traditionally believe that the spirit of the father's clan enters the baby early in pregnancy and the spirit of the mother's clan enters the baby at the naming ceremony, which takes place several months after birth.

Food Facts **Lemons**, like all citrus, are a great source of vitamin C during pregnancy. To get more juice from your lemon, bring it to room temperature or roll it between the heel of your hand and a hard surface, such as a countertop, before cutting. Meyer lemons are sweeter and less acidic than the common supermarket varieties.

Ask your child what he wants for dinner only if he's buying.
FRAN LEBOWITZ

DAY 91	DATE:
	175 days to go

At this point in development, your baby has a **considerable range of foot and leg movements:** Baby can kick, turn his or her feet outward and inward, and fan to curl his or her toes. If your baby is a boy, the male **prostate gland** has usually developed by now. The prostate contributes fluid that helps transport the sperm out of the adult male's body.

In another three or four weeks, **tiny stretch marks** (called striae gravidarum) may appear on your lower abdomen, buttocks, thighs, and breasts due to the rapid stretching of the skin. Stretch marks usually appear reddish or bluish at first; later they will fade to a silvery white.

Food Facts If cantaloupe and watermelon are available while you are pregnant, eat them, as they are good sources of both vitamins A and C. Most **melons** are also rich in natural folic acid. Interestingly, cantaloupe seeds are edible sources of omega-3 fat.

Did You Know? The hardest substance in your baby's body is tooth enamel.

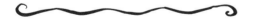

TIME TO REFLECT
What's the best advice you've received so far?

What do you want to be sure to remember?

(See page 84 for more space to write.)

Of all animals, the boy is the most unmanageable.
PLATO

Week 14 Begins

DAY 92	DATE:
	174 days to go

Rapid and sustained growth continues all this week. Over the next two days, your baby's **head and neck** will straighten as more bone is formed and the back muscles become stronger. **Slow eye movements begin under closed lids.** In two more weeks, baby's eyes will face forward.

You may experience occasional **nosebleeds and nasal stuffiness** due to increases in blood volume and the effects of the hormone estrogen, which causes your nasal membranes to swell.

Did You Know? If you do experience a **nosebleed**, applying pressure to the sides of the nose (about halfway down, past the bony tissue) probably works best to stop the bleeding. Sit upright and lean forward to avoid swallowing blood.

Childbirth Then and Now In England in the 1600s, pregnant women were expected to have unusual desires and cravings. The prevailing belief was that if a woman's desires were frustrated, their resulting anger could result in miscarriage. Thus, to prevent such problems, husbands were told by doctors to dote on their spouses.

Food Facts **Vitamins** are chemical compounds that are distinct from protein, carbohydrates, fats, and trace elements like iron. Because the body develops deficiency diseases without them, there are 13 vitamins essential to human health: A, B_1, B_2, B_6, B_{12}, C, D, E, K, niacin, folic acid and vitamin B_9, biotin (B_7), and pantothenic acid (B_5). Other substances may have nutrient value, but they don't belong on the list of vitamins.

DAY 93	DATE:
	173 days to go

Your baby's head and neck have assumed more of a straight-line relationship. Part of this repositioning might be due to the fact that the **skeleton is actively ossifying right now.**

Chances are you'll notice more **weight gain** during the next three months. It stands to reason that if your baby is growing rapidly, you should note some weight increases, too.

For Your Health Remember to **limit unnecessary or excess weight gain.** Extra weight will just be that much more difficult to lose after the baby is born, and also affects the baby's health.

Consider This **Vitamin B_2 (riboflavin) is a universal nutrient**, since small amounts of the vitamin are present in most plant and animal tissues. During pregnancy, the baby's body relies on riboflavin for normal cell growth, function, and energy production. Pregnant women need 27 percent more riboflavin—1.4 mg. Healthy, well-nourished individuals usually don't need supplemental B_2, since it can be obtained by drinking pasteurized milk and eating organic dairy products, fortified eggs, enriched whole grains and cereals, hormone-free meat, and organic broccoli and asparagus.

Childbirth Then and Now In 1639, in *An Alphabetical Book of Physical Secrets*, author Owen Woods suggested a pregnancy test: If a woman saw her reflection in her boiled urine, she was pregnant. (Whoa! Don't reuse *that* cookware!)

In youth we learn, in age we understand.
MARIE VON EBNER-ESCHENBACH

DAY 94	DATE:
	172 days to go

During this month, your baby's **body will begin to grow faster than his or her head.**

You may notice that some clear fluid can be expressed from your breasts— this is not colostrum (a yellowish fluid rich in protein and antibodies), which won't appear until the end of Week 16. It is fluid that has accumulated in your mammary glands due to the changing levels of hormones in your system. Interestingly, while the breasts of an adult woman look mature, women's breasts don't finish developing until they prepare for milk production during pregnancy!

Food Facts **Vitamin A is essential.** It regulates cell growth and cell division. It plays a role in fighting infection and maintaining the health of the hair, skin, mucous membranes like those that line the nose, and the cells that line the inner surfaces of the body. Vitamin A also promotes the growth of bones and teeth and is necessary for dim light vision. Although **natural Vitamin A is found only in foods of animal origin**, some fruits and vegetables like carrots contain compounds that can be converted into vitamin A. The liver stores 90 percent of the body's vitamin A—a 6- to 12-month supply.

For Your Information **By this time, your baby's external genitals are distinctly male or distinctly female in appearance.**

Childbirth in Other Cultures Historically, Native American women and their newborns plunged into a stream immediately after delivery. If a stream wasn't available, the child was dipped in cold water as soon as it was born. Saltwater baths and washes were used by people who lived by the sea. The cold-water bath was considered to be an initiation of the newborn child into the troubles of this world.

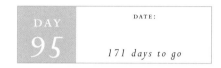

DAY 95	DATE:
	171 days to go

Over the next three days, your **baby's toenails** will begin to grow from their nail beds. Baby's **legs** have lengthened and have functional joints.

Nasal congestion is common during pregnancy as the mucous membranes swell. You may feel particularly congested during the winter months, when dry, heated air circulates to warm the house, or if you have a cold; you also may be uncomfortable when it's warmer and allergies compound nasal stuffiness. Your ears may also feel full or stuffy.

If the full sensation in your nose or ears is accompanied by pain, fever, or flulike symptoms, **check with your practitioner to make sure you don't have an infection.** If you are running a temperature, your baby's environment warms up, too. Consult with your practitioner before you take anything for symptom relief.

Consider This **A natural way to reduce nasal congestion is to use saline**, either as a nasal spray or a nasal wash. Check any other over-the-counter remedies with your practitioner.

Food Facts **Avoid eating liver** during pregnancy. It contains high levels of vitamin A; the liver's function is to screen impurities out of the body and neutralize toxins, so naturally it's full of things to be avoided.

Teach your child to hold his tongue. He'll learn fast enough to speak.
BENJAMIN FRANKLIN

TIME TO REFLECT

Are you hoping for a son or a daughter or just a healthy baby?

....

....

....

....

....

limit their caffeine intake to the equivalent of 1 cup of coffee per day. **Once again, err on the side of caution and give up caffeine altogether.**

Chart your waist size and weight here and on page 181.

WAIST SIZE WEIGHT

DAY
96

DATE:

170 days to go

Even though the baby draws heavily from the nutrients in your bloodstream, **there's always something left for your system.** ☺
As the **ligaments that support your uterus** stretch, you may experience back and/or abdominal pain.

Did You Know? You may be **more comfortable** sitting rather than standing. To help reduce pain, keep your knees spread wide apart while standing up from a chair or bed. In addition, warm baths and the heat generated by a heating pad might warm the abdominal and lower back muscles enough to relax them and provide some relief. Avoid hot tubs and saunas that could raise your core body temperarture to 102°F (39°C) or above.

Food Facts The caffeine from any source (coffee, tea, soda, energy drinks, and cocoa) seems to encourage the uterus to contract. Pregnant women are urged to

---

DAY
97

DATE:

169 days to go

Your baby's head now appears upright—the **chin** no longer seems to rest on the chest. The **ears** are close to their final position. The **toenails** are growing from their nail beds.

As your uterus shifts and relieves pressure from your bladder, you may find you don't have to urinate quite as frequently. **Enjoy it while it lasts!** Toward the end of your pregnancy, frequent urination will return. You might want to carry tissue and toilet seat covers with you in your purse, pack, or car in case you need to stop at facilities that are less than sanitary. Also, continue to take steps to avoid constipation.

Consider This You'll probably feel most comfortable now that you're in your second trimester. With any luck, morning sickness (if you had it) may be past and your energy level is likely to be up. This may be a good time to take a family vacation or plan some activities with your older child before the new baby comes. **Your energy level and equilibrium might shift again around Week 25, when your third trimester starts.**

Where we love is home, home that the feet may leave, but not our hearts.

OLIVER WENDELL HOLMES

Food Facts **The peel on fruits like bananas, melons, and oranges is not an absolute barrier** to pesticides, herbicides, and chemical fertilizers used when the fruit was grown. Eat organically grown fruit whenever possible.

Childbirth in Other Cultures The Luzon of the Philippines believe that if an expectant mother quarrels with her own mother or with her mother-in-law, she will have a difficult delivery.

What do you want to be sure to remember?

(See page 84 for more space to write.)

DAY 98	DATE:
	168 days to go

Your baby is the size of a thick 5-inch candy bar—4¾ inches long (120 mm) crown to rump and weighs 3¾ oz (104.5 g), having **more than doubled his or her dimensions** in a mere two weeks.

You may notice that your veins are becoming more apparent because of the extra volume of blood created by your system to support the pregnancy. **The average amount of blood lost during a completely normal birth is about one pint,** or the amount that is given when donating one unit of blood.

Did You Know? Some **nutrients play critical roles** in basic metabolism. For example, magnesium helps regulate insulin and blood-sugar levels and influences cholesterol, while potassium helps release energy stored in foods containing protein, fat, and carbohydrates.

Food Facts Lettuce and other salad greens should be washed well before they are eaten but never soaked, since **soaking extracts the vitamins.** Iceberg lettuce is mostly water, but organically grown romaine lettuce is loaded with nutrition. The greener the lettuce leaf, the more nutrition it provides.

The hardest job kids face today is learning good manners without seeing any.

FRED ASTAIRE

LMP Week 17

DAY 99	DATE:
	167 days to go

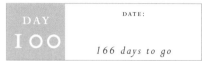 **During this entire week, the baby grows rapidly**, with growth setting the stage for development later this month. Your baby's weight will increase six times during this fourth month of pregnancy. Even then, the baby will only weigh 6 oz (168 g), not even half a pound.

You probably still feel tired and some-times out of energy. That's normal. Plenty of rest, high-quality nutrition, and exercise should make you feel better. Exercise doesn't have to be a full workout—5 to 10 minutes of walking, stretching, yoga, or other activity is renewing (when you can find the energy to do it!). If you have chil-dren at home, try to rest when they do or get some-one you trust to watch them while you lie down.

Childbirth Then and Now To hurry her labor, the Klamath Indian woman would tell her baby that a rattlesnake was coming to bite him, if he did not hurry out of the womb!

Food Facts When **fruit is dried**, about 50 percent of the water is removed, but sugar may be added, especially to cranberries, pineapple, and bananas. Dried apples are often lower in calories than other choices.

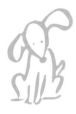

DAY 100	DATE:
	166 days to go

Blood travels with considerable force through the **umbilical cord**, giving the cord the same kind of tension as a water-filled hose. The cord resists knotting and tends to straighten itself out as your baby moves about.

If you're **feeling faint or woozy**, it's possible that you're not eating properly or are dehydrated, especially if you're running after a toddler or trying to juggle a busy schedule. Sit or lie down to stabilize yourself first, and then eat a healthy snack and drink some water. Keep nutritious snacks and water close at hand—in your purse, your car, and in your toddler's diaper bag or your older child's backpack. It's also possible that you might be feeling overheated. Wear layers of clothing you can peel off when you need to.

If you will be pregnant during **cold and flu season**, talk to your health-care provider about getting a flu shot. **Changes in your immune system during pregnancy make you more vulnerable to illness and infection, not less.** Wash your hands frequently and stay well rested. Keep the rest of your family as healthy as you can, and when you're out, avoid crowds.

Did You Know? The baby's link to the placenta is the **umbilical cord.** The umbilical cord usually extends from the center of the placenta, but it may be located anywhere on the placenta's surface.

Children need love, especially when they do not deserve it.

HAROLD S. HULBERT

DAY	DATE:
101	165 days to go

With the help of the placenta and the umbilical cord, **your baby's system is operating as it will after birth.** The baby has his or her own circulation, pumped by the heart, which at this developmental stage pumps the equivalent of 25 qt of blood (27.5 l) a day. The placenta helps with disease protection, digestion, oxygenation, waste removal, and hormone production. Most bacteria are unable to pass through the placental membrane, but most drugs and medications cross the placenta freely.

The chances are good that you've noticed an **increase in your appetite.** Eating nutritious food provides fuel to sustain the baby's growth and to give you the energy you need to manage all the "nonpregnant" aspects of your life.

Childbirth Then and Now Rural birth attendants in pioneer America were often neighbors and grannies. Their advice following childbirth: "Eat anything y'want except kraut and pickled beans, and stay in th'bed for ten days."

Food Facts The **development of the baby's brain cells** is particularly dependent on available protein and heart-healthy fats. Biotin, or vitamin B_7, is needed to manufacture fats, proteins, and glycogen essential to brain and liver function. The recommended daily intake of biotin during pregnancy is 30 mcg. Primary sources of biotin include whole grains, dried beans, nuts, cooked eggs, and cauliflower.

DAY	DATE:
102	164 days to go

Your baby is getting bigger this week. Baby is also adding to his or her list of **reflex behaviors**. Reflexes are the automatic, unlearned behaviors a baby is born with. Most reflexes have survival value for infants: Blinking helps keep foreign objects out of their eyes and keeps their eyes moist; sucking and swallowing permit nourishment. Right now, your baby is practicing all three of these reflex behaviors. He or she is also working on incorporating some additional reflexes, so that by the time he or she is born, the average full-term baby will display more than 70 different reflex behaviors.

During this month, the **placenta** will become the main source of hormones needed to sustain the pregnancy and to prepare for the production of milk. Later, the placenta will play an important role in determining the changing hormone balance that will help to initiate labor and birth.

Childbirth in Other Cultures To the Jarawa of the Andaman Islands off India, childbirth is such a normal event that it traditionally takes place in full view of everyone.

Food Facts Choline is an essential B vitamin found in these natural foods: egg yolk, organic oats, sesame seeds, flaxseed, peanuts, potatoes, soybeans, cauliflower, lentils, pork loin, roasted chicken, ground beef, and shrimp. Preliminary research findings suggest that **choline influences brain growth** by producing bigger cells in vital brain areas involved in memory and muscle control. The recommended daily intake of choline during pregnancy is 450 mg.

Every beetle is a gazelle in the eyes of its mother.
MOORISH PROVERB

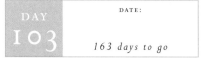

Chart your waist size and weight here and on page 181.

WAIST SIZE   WEIGHT

DAY **103**   DATE:

163 days to go

Sometime this week, your baby's **kidneys** will reach their final mature position. This ascent took nearly 10 weeks to complete because the body had to straighten to bring the kidneys into the abdomen. **Body straightening** is only one part of this month's astounding growth. For example, your baby grows so much that he or she reaches half the length measured at birth!

Private non-diagnostic 3-D/4-D ultrasound portraiture or video of your baby is becoming increasingly available. The procedure is fee-based and may or may not be performed by a registered sonographer. The timing of the sonogram makes a difference. When the baby is younger, you'll get to see more of them, but less detail is visible. When the baby is older, you'll get to see more detail, but less of them. Alternatively, wait until your baby is born to see all of them in complete detail— for free!

Food Facts If you don't care for plain **broccoli**, it can easily be included in soups, salads, healthy stir-fries, stews, omelets, quiche, and potato dishes. Although it's a sulfur-containing vegetable, fresh broccoli smells sweet.

DAY **104**   DATE:

162 days to go

During this month, the baby and the **placenta** are nearly equal in size, but the baby will soon grow larger than the placenta. The placenta performs the functions that the baby's digestive system, lungs, and kidneys will provide after birth.

As your baby grows larger and stronger, it becomes more and more likely that you'll actually begin to feel him or her move. At first the baby feels like a butterfly fluttering in your abdomen. The very earliest movements are reported around Week 14 or 15. More likely, **you will feel your baby move at the same time as the majority of women do: sometime around Week 18, 19, or 20.**

Did You Know? Worldwide, competent midwives decrease the risk of lives lost during childbirth. The word **midwife** comes from Old English words meaning "with the woman" (*mid* = with and *wif* = woman). Similarly, in Latin, the midwife is the *cummater*, and in Portuguese and Spanish, she is the *comadre*. Among the ancient Jews, she is the "wise woman," a characterization reflected both in the modern German term, *weise frau*, and in the modern French, *sage-femme*.

Food Facts The recommended daily value for **vitamin A** intake during pregnancy is 970 IU. Because of its potential for liver damage, vitamin A needs are best met through foods, not dietary supplements. Vitamin A in the form of natural carotenoids (like beta-carotene in carrots) does not seem harmful. Cooked, canned pumpkin and cooked sweet potatoes are excellent sources.

Definition: fairy tale, n. A horror story to prepare children for newspapers.
AMBROSE BIERCE

DAY 105	DATE:
	161 days to go

This was a week of **rapid, whole-body growth** for your baby. Existing structures became larger and more well developed, but no new structures were formed.

The chances are good that this week's growth spurt for your baby also resulted in a **growth spurt for you.**

Food Facts **Fresh potatoes** are rich in vitamin C. One medium baked or roasted potato yields 29 mg of the vitamin (more than 25 percent of your day's requirement), more potassium than a banana, and more than 10 percent of the fiber needed daily, primarily in the skin. Potatoes have phytonutrients that resemble the profile for broccoli and spinach, along with antioxidant and heart-healthy benefits. In its unadulterated form—not fried (healthy stir-fry is okay) or slathered with butter and sour cream—the potato can easily become a low-calorie dietary mainstay. But as French fries or potato chips eaten on a weekly basis, potatoes have been linked to unhealthy weight gain, breast cancer, diabetes, and heart problems due to high levels of fat, calories, and salt.

Childbirth in Other Cultures If a baby girl is born to a Mayan woman living in the Yucatán Peninsula, the mother traditionally has her baby's ears pierced before she is 60 minutes old. Mayans believe that babies don't feel anything so soon after birth; a day later, she would be "paying attention."

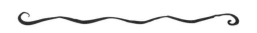

TIME TO REFLECT
What has surprised you most so far about your pregnancy?

What do you want to be sure to remember?

(See page 84 for more space to write.)

Level with your child by being honest. Nobody spots a phony quicker than a child.
MARY MACCRACKEN

LMP Week 18

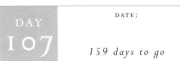

DAY 106	DATE:
	160 days to go

DAY 107	DATE:
	159 days to go

By now, all the major elements of the **lungs** have formed except those involved with the oxygen–carbon dioxide exchange; breathing air is not yet possible. Over the next three days, pads will begin to form on your baby's **fingertips and toes.**

A thin, whitish **vaginal discharge** called leukorrhea is normally secreted during pregnancy. You may notice this secretion becoming heavier as your pregnancy continues.

Contact your practitioner if the vaginal discharge changes color (becomes yellowish or greenish), thickens, or is accompanied by burning, itching, or pain during urination. These symptoms may require attention.

Did You Know? The early development of the placenta is actually directed by **chromosomes contributed by the father's sperm, not the mother's egg.**

Food Facts **Reduce your exposure to toxins:**
1. Store and eat from food in glass rather than plastic dishes. 2. Don't assume that your ceramic pottery pieces are necessarily food-safe. 3. Avoid cookware and cooking utensils with plastic handles; if they overheat and start to melt, they can release toxic fumes.

By today, the early solid waste material called **meconium** will begin to accumulate in your baby's bowel. This material is the product of cell turnover, digestive secretions, and swallowed amniotic fluid and is the result of the digestive system practicing digestion while still in the womb. For the most part, swallowed amniotic fluid is absorbed by the intestine and directed toward the placental membrane into the maternal blood for elimination by the mother's kidneys.

Your carbohydrate needs will increase during these last two trimesters of pregnancy. Carbohydrates provide your body with energy and can be found in sugars, starches, and fiber.

Food Facts **Canned vegetables and fruits** are higher in carbohydrates than fresh vegetables and fruits, because the canning process can add refined sugar to the natural sugars already found in these foods.

For Your Health: Even though exposure to peanuts, milk, and wheat gluten during the first trimester can strengthen your child's immune system, you might consider **avoiding those foods during your third trimester.** Ironically, exposure toward the end of your pregnancy can increase your baby's chances of developing asthma and allergies to these foods.

You didn't have a choice about the parents you inherited, but you do have a choice about the kind of parent you will be.

MARIAN WRIGHT EDELMAN

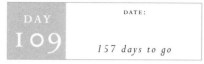

DAY 108	DATE:
	158 days to go

By today, your baby has pads on his or her fingertips and toes that will develop the characteristic swirls and creases of the **finger- and toeprints.**

As you identify yourself more and more with being pregnant, you might find that even if you're excited about having a baby, you sometimes feel scared, worried, or ambivalent about the future. You should know that **pregnancy is a mix of both positive and negative feelings** and that your particular feelings are perfectly normal. While worry cannot help by itself, being worried about the future might help you plan and solve problems that take some of the guesswork out of adjusting to a new baby. Don't worry if you don't have all the answers—no one does. The good news is that you've got questions, and you can find answers if you just ask. Physicians, midwives, lactation consultants, friends, parents, authors, organizations, and counselors are all good resources. There's also lots of information online.

Food Facts If you need a **quick pick-me-up beverage**, avoid soda, coffee, and energy drinks. Instead, try organic vegetable juice, unsweetened diluted natural fruit juice, diluted citrus juice (if you can tolerate citrus), or water with natural lemon or lime.

DAY 109	DATE:
	157 days to go

Your **baby's eyes** now look forward rather than to the side.

While the **placenta** serves to keep the baby healthy, it also plays a role in safeguarding your health. The placenta can synthesize natural ingredients in the blood that prevent infection. While most of these **infection-fighters** are dispensed to the baby, you receive some as well, especially during the last three months of pregnancy. Great teamwork!

Food Facts **Vitamin C** is a nutrient that works in concert with zinc, iron, and vitamin E, but it's also powerful on its own. Vitamin C seems to protect us against viruses, heart disease, the accumulation of lead in our tissues, environmental tobacco smoke, and developing cataracts (with vitamin E). This **super-vitamin** also helps detoxify alcohol, makes collagen to keep muscles strong and blood vessels supple, heals wounds, repairs damaged cells in the arteries of the heart, and protects the eyes, nerves, and kidneys of people with diabetes!

Childbirth Then and Now In colonial America, it was common to have the laboring woman seated on her husband's lap, he being seated on a chair. He would hold onto the woman around the top of her abdomen or under her arms. As a male writer commented in 1882:

> This position was certainly not a bad one for all parties with the exception of the husband who, in tedious cases, suffered rather severely; but then this little tax on his affectionate nature was, in those days, considered the very least return he could make for the mischief he had occasioned.

I have found that the best way to give advice to your children is to find out what they want and then to advise them to do it.

HARRY S. TRUMAN

DAY 110	DATE:
	156 days to go

Over the next two days, the **ears** will move to their final positions. The **major glands** in the hormone-producing endocrine system include the pituitary, pineal, thyroid, adrenal, kidneys, liver, pancreas, and ovaries or testes. Most endocrine glands secrete hormones that appear in the baby's bloodstream as early as Week 12, but certainly by Week 20.

From this week on, **your heart** has to work 40 to 50 percent harder to support your pregnancy. Generally, this added workload doesn't pose a problem—a healthy heart can cope with the increased demand.

Talk to your practitioner about habit management or treatment options for smoking and drinking. They're here to help.

IMPORTANT: There's no amount of alcohol or number of tobacco or marijuana cigarettes that's safe during pregnancy.

Did You Know? According to the Centers for Disease Control, about 10,773 babies are born each day in the United States.

Chart your waist size and weight here and on page 181.

WAIST SIZE   WEIGHT

DAY 111	DATE:
	155 days to go

Many of your baby's bones have begun to harden, **making them visible** in ultrasound images.

After you have a meal, your baby receives its nutrients within an hour or two.

Did You Know? Your baby will be **born with 300 bones** in its body. As your child grows, some bones will fuse together to produce a total of 206 bones by adulthood.

Food Facts Consider using **fresh organic seasonings** like garlic, onion, shallots, lemongrass, and juice from lemons or limes when you cook. Try some naturally flavored salts on your favorite dishes.

Childbirth in Other Cultures Soranus, a Greek physician who lived in the second century CE, would be the equivalent of a modern ob-gyn. He described the ideal midwife as a woman of a sympathetic disposition (although she need not have borne a child herself), endowed with slim fingers with short nails at the fingertips, who keeps her hands soft for the comfort of both the mother and the child. Excellent!

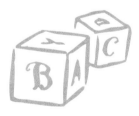

Who takes the child by the hand takes the mother by the heart.
GERMAN PROVERB

DAY 112

DATE:

154 days to go

Sometime during this, week the process of myelinization begins. **Myelinization** involves coating the nerves with a fatty substance (called myelin) to speed nerve cell transmission and to insulate the nerves so messages are uninterrupted. The baby that has been growing so rapidly inside you now measures 5½ inches (140 mm) in length, big enough for you to cradle in the palm of your hand!

By now you may have felt your baby's fluttery movement for the first time! The baby has been moving steadily. If you haven't yet felt the movement, you most likely will during these next two weeks. Again, don't expect bumps and thumps right now. The feelings will be more like a growling stomach, a bubble bursting, butterflies in the stomach—even indigestion or hunger pains.

Food Facts **Natural cheese** is a good food choice during pregnancy because it is a concentrated source of many of the nutrients found in milk. The protein obtained from cheese is of equal quality to meat protein, usually costs much less, and keeps animals alive.

Did You Know? **Cheese varies considerably in terms of calcium content.** For example, 60 grams of feta cheese has 270 mg of calcium and is great on vegetables or salad. It takes twice the amount of soft cheese—like Brie—to equal the amount of calcium in a hard cheese like cheddar or Parmesan. Select natural cheese made from pasteurized products and stay away from processed cheese.

What do you want to be sure to remember?

(See page 84 for more space to write.)

TIME TO REFLECT
What are you especially excited about right now?

Feel the dignity of a child. Do not feel superior to him, for you are not.
ROBERT HENRI

*What do you want to remember about your **Fourth Month**?*

Lunar Month 5

THINGS TO DO THIS MONTH:

* Acknowledge any ambivalent feelings; do what you can to adjust.

* Pamper yourself—you'll also be pampering your baby.

* Try to gain only healthy weight.

* Wear comfortable, layered clothing so you can add or subtract as needed.

* Eat locally grown food whenever possible.

* Manage back pain with postural changes, controlling weight gain, and proper footwear.

* Limit fast food, processed food, foods high in refined sugar, and unhealthy fats.

* Drink decaffeinated beverages.

* Continue to lie on your left side and use pillows to support your legs and abdomen.

* Increase your intake of high-density lipoproteins (HDLs) to manage your cholesterol.

* Check with your practitioner about the safety of spa, hair, nail, and other salon treatments.

* Check with your dentist if you have severe gum pain or discomfort or are considering a whitening treatment or oral surgery.

Week 17 Begins

LMP Week 19

DAY 113	DATE: 153 days to go

Your baby's **external ears** now stand out from his or her head. Over this next month, your baby will gain about 2 inches (51 mm) in height and more than a pound-and-a-half (26 oz or 728 g) in weight.

Congratulations, you've now been pregnant for four months! **In two more weeks, you'll be halfway to your baby's birthdate!**

Think About It **Whether your pregnancy is going quickly or slowly doesn't matter as much as whether it's going well.** Remember— you are building your baby cell by cell. **Pampering yourself actually means pampering your baby**; don't feel selfish if you need extra rest time, choose to cut down on activities, or indulge in a massage.

Childbirth in Other Cultures While many cultures prescribe that only women can assist a laboring woman, the Lepcha of the Himalayas express no gender preference: Any knowledgeable person can attend the birth and help the mother.

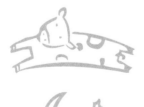

DAY 114	DATE: 152 days to go

Over the next two days, **temporary downy hair** (lanugo) will begin to appear on your baby's head and body. The lanugo helps hold a protective coating called vernix on the skin, and by the time the baby is born, most of the lanugo will have disappeared.

You'll gain most of your weight in the next three months. Generally, you might expect an average increase of a pound a week until Month 7. Weight gain will be mostly uneven, though. It's much more common to gain nothing one week, 2 lb (907 g) the next, ½ lb (227 g) the following week, and so on. Continue eating high-quality nutrients so you're gaining healthy weight. Take care not to get too tired, since the rapid growth of the baby this month will require your heart, lungs, and kidneys to work much harder.

Food Facts Calcium; phosphorus; vitamins C, D, and K; magnesium; zinc; manganese; and fluoride **build your baby's bones and teeth.** Even though fresh organic vegetables are generally poor sources of calcium compared to milk and milk products, cooked dark-green leafy vegetables (especially kale, collard greens, and spinach) do offer significant amounts.

Did You Know? Percent Daily Values (%DV) of specific nutrients were first established by the National Academy of Sciences in 1941 in response to concerns about **deficiency diseases in men serving in World War II and the health of U.S. citizens** living back in the States with food in short supply.

Children in families are like flowers in a bouquet:
there's always one determined to face in an opposite direction from the way the arranger desires.
MARCELENE COX

| DAY 115 | DATE:
151 days to go |
|---|---|

Last month, your baby grew from 3½ inches (89 mm) long to 5½ inches (140 mm) long. That's a **substantial size increase.** This month, growth slows somewhat, but the results are still dramatic. In four short weeks, your baby will grow from 5½ inches (140 mm) in length to 8 to 10 inches (203 to 254 mm) long!

As you gain more weight, you may want to switch to fuller, less-restrictive clothing made from lighter weight, natural fabrics. This will keep you more comfortable as **your body temperature increases.**

Food Facts Organically grown **corn** is a good source of pregnancy-supporting vitamins and fiber. Since the sugar in the kernels begins to turn to starch immediately after harvesting, the best source for fresh corn is a local farmers' market. Do not remove the husks until just before cooking. Three minutes in boiling water sets the milk in the corn that is rich in flavor and nutrients. Do not salt the water, as this tends to harden the kernels. Corn can also be cooked on the grill or in the microwave.

Childbirth in Other Cultures Traditionally, most West African tribal cultures believe that a baby is so close to the spirit world that both the baby and mother are vulnerable to the influence of evil spirits. For protection, the mother is told to wear special amulets and charms and to avoid doing anything that would attract the attention of the spirits.

Chart your waist size and weight here and on page 181.

WAIST SIZE   WEIGHT

| DAY 116 | DATE:
150 days to go |
|---|---|

If your baby is a girl, miniature egg cells—about 2 million of them—now exist in her ovaries. Although women may make new eggs over time, by the time your daughter is ready to have a family of her own, most of her eggs will be as old as she is!

If you haven't had back pain yet, you may notice it as your pregnancy continues. Most pregnancy backaches consist of low back pain, because the narrowest part of your back (your waist) has to balance your growing uterus and because the normally stable joints in your pelvis have loosened somewhat. Since backache is so common during pregnancy, over the next week or so, I'll list nine suggestions, one at a time, for avoiding or minimizing backache.

NO MORE ACHING BACK *Suggestion #1:* **Maintain good posture.** Pretend there is a string running through your backbone and out the top of your head. Imagine being pulled up by the string. Align your head, neck, backbone, and pelvis. Feel yourself lift and straighten. Consciously straighten your alignment when you feel yourself slouch, keeping weight evenly on both feet, which are a comfortable distance apart. Keep your pelvis under you, not tipped forward. Yoga and stretching may also help.

For there is no kind that had any other first beginning. For all men have one entrance into life.
THE WISDOM OF SOLOMON IN THE APOCRYPHA

Childbirth in Other Cultures By tradition, Hopi women of the American Southwest are encouraged to get up early every morning and not to sit around during pregnancy. The Sanpoil tribe goes even further. For their pregnant woman, a regular program of exercise, mainly walking and swimming in the nearby Columbia River (U.S. state of Washington), is prescribed.

Childbirth in Other Cultures A custom among the nineteenth-century Loango of Africa was that as long as the umbilical stump was still on the child, no male being, not even the father, would be admitted into the presence of the newborn for fear that the child would fall into evil ways.

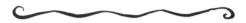

DAY 117	DATE:
	149 days to go

Over the next two days, the **vernix** begins to form. This is a creamy-looking substance that covers your baby's skin in order to protect it and its developing glands and sensory cells. The vernix is composed of dead skin, oil from the oil-bearing glands of the baby's skin, and the lanugo.

By this time, you may have noticed the appearance of a mottled area of pigmentation that extends beyond the existing nipple and areola and sometimes covers half of the breast. Called the **secondary areola**, this pigmentation change in breast tissue is temporary, but it may last for as long as twelve months after the birth.

NO MORE ACHING BACK *Suggestion #2:*
Avoid extra weight gain. The more additional weight you put on, the more weight your back will have to balance. If you cut out all of the fast food, processed food, and other foods high in fat and sugar, any weight you gain will be "healthy weight."

TIME TO REFLECT
What sounds good to you right now?

What do you want to be sure to remember?

(See page 102 for more space to write.)

Children are remarkable for their intelligence and ardor, for their curiosity, their intolerance of shams, the clarity and ruthlessness of their vision.

ALDOUS HUXLEY

DAY 118

DATE:

148 days to go

The **vernix** has begun to form over your baby's entire body.

In addition to breast changes, blotchy areas of pigmentation may appear on your forehead and on the sides of your face. This pigmentation is called the **mask of pregnancy** (chloasma). Because exposure to the sun can darken the area and make it less likely to fade, continue to use a facial sunscreen daily. Any pigmentation changes usually fade within a few months of childbirth.

NO MORE ACHING BACK *Suggestion #3:*

When you sit, elevate your legs on a footstool or stretch out on the couch to take the pressure off your back. Avoid standing or sitting too long in one position. Asymmetrical positions (like supporting one leg on a stool while standing) can sometimes worsen joint pain.

Childbirth Then and Now "Two or three years ago (1879–1880), an Indian party of Flat Heads and Kootenais men, women, and children, set out for a hunting trip. On a severely cold winter's day in the Rocky Mountains, one of the women, allowing the party to proceed, dismounted from her horse, spread an old buffalo robe upon the snow and gave birth to a child which was immediately followed by the placenta. Having attended to everything as well as the circumstances permitted, she wrapped up the young one in a blanket, mounted her horse, and overtook the party before they had noticed her absence." **Women are amazing!** (Engelmann, *Labor Among Primitive Peoples*, 1882)

DAY 119

DATE:

147 days to go

From now until your baby is born, the **placenta** will grow in diameter but not in thickness. Ultimately, it will grow to over 8 inches (22 cm) in diameter. The word **placenta** comes from the Greek for "flat cake."

Occasionally, the baby will hiccup, causing a rhythmic jarring of your abdomen every two to four seconds or so. While there is no air to intake, hiccuping in the womb involves the same sort of muscular reactions as in an air-breathing child. The hiccuping generally stops in about a half hour. By the time you go to bed tonight, you will have been pregnant for eighteen weeks—4½ whole months!

For Your Information One of the biggest **lifting challenges** will be getting your other children in and out of the tub while you're pregnant. Using the bathtub involves a lot of awkward positioning. It may be easier and safer to bathe the children in the sink or fill a tub on the kitchen counter.

Food Facts While naturally produced meats, cheeses, and eggs add saturated **fats** to your diet during pregnancy, the fat portion of organic nuts and seeds is highly unsaturated and is better for your brain, heart, and arteries. Coconuts are the exception—they're high in saturated fats and not a good source of protein.

Whatever you are, be a good one.
WILLIAM MAKEPEACE THACKERAY

LMP Week 20

DAY 120	DATE:
	146 days to go

DAY 121	DATE:
	145 days to go

By today, heat-producing **brown fat begins to form** at the base of your baby's neck, by the breastbone, and near the urethra—the tube that passes urine out of the body. Brown fat has a protective function: It helps keep the baby warm in cold environments. Brown fat exists in newborns, but it tends to diminish with age.

If you have darker hair or skin, the pigmentation of the white line between your navel and pubic bone or **linea alba** generally becomes darkly pigmented during pregnancy.

NO MORE ACHING BACK *Suggestion #4:*
Wear shoes that give your feet stability and support. Some heel is actually better than no heel at all, but don't go over 2 inches—you might lose your balance and fall. Consider investing in a good pair of walking shoes. A wide variety of footwear and insoles are specifically designed for pregnancy.

Food Facts **Omega-3 fatty acids are healthy fats.** Food sources include fatty fish like salmon, sardines, herring, and cod. Nutritionists advise eating one or more sources of omega-3 fats each day.

Over the next two days, your baby's **eyebrows** will begin to form. Eyebrows and head hair are visible by 20 weeks.

Your pituitary gland is responsible for the **pigmentation changes** you see in your skin. It releases more melanin or pigment-stimulating hormone during pregnancy than when you're not pregnant, and more melanin if you have darker skin or hair than if you are naturally lighter.

NO MORE ACHING BACK *Suggestion #5:*
If you have to lift something, first make sure it's not too heavy, then **lift with your legs—not with your back.** Bend at your knees, keeping your back fairly straight, grasp the object, then straighten your legs to lift. If you can get into the habit of lifting with your legs, you'll protect yourself from back injury and strain even when you aren't pregnant. If you are pushing a stroller, make sure the handles are at a comfortable height.

Food Facts Since you are strongly advised to limit your caffeinated coffee intake, you will want to have the **tastiest coffee** you can when you treat yourself to an occasional cup. There are many excellent coffeehouses to choose from or you may want to brew your own. The essential flavoring in coffee comes from caffeol, a substance that is lost by exposure to air. In order for caffeol to be released, the beans must be freshly ground.

Raising a child is like reading a very long mystery story;
you have to wait for a generation to see how it turns out.
ANONYMOUS

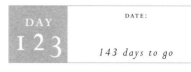

DAY **122**	DATE:
	144 days to go

The baby sleeps and wakes as much as a newborn does now. When your baby sleeps, he or she characteristically settles into a favorite position or "lie." Some babies always sleep with their chins resting on the chest, while others tilt their heads back.

NO MORE ACHING BACK *Suggestion #6:*
Try to avoid carrying objects or babies in your arms while pregnant. Weight in your arms only adds to the weight already out in front of you. Carry objects down at your sides, use a tote with wheels, or ask for help.

Did You Know? The **plaque** or coating on the inside of the walls of the heart and arteries is the same plaque that coats brain cells, interferes with their function, and may lead to the development of Alzheimer's disease.

Childbirth Then and Now The custom among the West Micronesians on the Isle of Yap during the nineteenth century was to begin to dilate a pregnant woman's cervix at least one month before delivery was expected. The leaves of a certain plant were rolled into a tight tube and inserted into the cervix. When dilated to that size, a thicker roll was introduced. This pre-labor dilation of the cervix made labor faster and less painful, but the procedure itself caused some cramping and discomfort.

DAY **123**	DATE:
	143 days to go

Over the next three days, **fine scalp hair will start to form** on your baby's head. (This is the permanent hair, not lanugo.) Even this "permanent hair" will begin to fall out in the second week following birth, to be replaced gradually by coarser, thicker hair.

NO MORE ACHING BACK *Suggestion #7:*
Ask your practitioner about **exercises to strengthen and maintain your back muscles** or do something you're already competent at, like walking, stretching, or swimming.

Childbirth Then and Now The **obstetric chair**— a chair with a back and false bottom—was first developed for use in Europe in the 1540s, but the original design dates back to the earliest known papyrus records from ancient Egypt. The chair is still in use today.

Food Facts As beneficial as protein is now that you're pregnant, **too much protein could be as harmful as too little.** Stay within the recommended dietary guidelines (no more than 100 grams daily) and consult with your practitioner about adjustments.

A happy childhood can't be cured. Mine'll hang around my neck like a rainbow.
HORTENSE CALISHER

TIME TO REFLECT
What do you find yourself doing with your free time?

_____

_____

_____

_____

DAY 124	DATE:
	142 days to go

In the next three days, the vernix becomes noticeable on your **baby's skin.**

From Week 12 to Week 20, the placenta weighs as much as, if not more than, the baby, because **it has to work hard** to extract the nutrients from food and dispose of waste. The fetal organs are not sufficiently mature to digest food.

NO MORE ACHING BACK *Suggestion #8:*
Try a professional pregnancy **massage** or ask a partner to use their thumb or knuckle to press the spot that's especially sore gently but deeply for 1 to 2 minutes.

Food Facts **Your baby's body needs fat for proper development and tissue maintenance.** Fat coats the nerve cells in the brain and spinal cord to speed the transmission of information from one part of the nervous system to the other. Fat stores and releases energy, and it also helps control what gets in and out of cells. It's so important that even so-called diet foods like carrots and lettuce contain small amounts

of fat. The key to understanding fat is understanding what type of fat it is—that is, whether it's good for your health or bad.

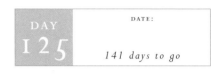

DAY 125	DATE:
	141 days to go

By today, hair will have begun to form on your baby's head. **In another month, the head hair may be up to an inch long on a head that's about the size of a tangerine.**

You may sleep more comfortably if you lie on your left side with **a pillow** between your knees to keep your thighs parallel to the bed. This support will keep your upper leg from falling to the mattress and aggravating back pain. Also, place a pillow under your abdomen to take the weight off your lower back. A full-body pillow may be useful.

Food Facts **Good fats are good for your heart and brain.** Healthy fats come from fish, organic vegetables, tree nuts, and seeds. When extracted from their food sources, these good fats are liquid (i.e., unsaturated) at room temperature so that they can move around the body freely. Unhealthy fats can coat and clog because they are solid (i.e., saturated) at room temperature. **Bad fats and oils** come mainly from all types of red meat, seafood, dairy (ice cream), fast foods, and some restaurant foods like baked goods and French fries.

Did You Know? **Cholesterol** is a fat that is carried in the bloodstream by special proteins called lipoproteins. Regarding heart and brain health, there are low-density lipoproteins (LDL), which carry cholesterol from the liver or bloodstream and deposit it to form plaques on brain cells, the heart, and arteries,

---

The best way to keep children home is to make the home atmosphere pleasant—and let the air out of the tires.
DOROTHY PARKER

and high-density lipoproteins (HDL), which try to collect as much cholesterol as possible from the bloodstream, from LDL, and from arteries and cells and take it to the liver to be destroyed. In other words, **LDL is HDL's evil twin.**

Childbirth Then and Now In the 1800s, inhabitants of the island of Ceram, north of Australia, tied laboring women to a post or tree with their hands above their heads. Often, the woman was semisuspended. This practice seemed to cut labor time—so that women could return to their responsibilities sooner.

DAY 126	DATE: *140 days to go*

By this time, if your baby is a girl, her uterus has completely formed and the vagina, hymen, and labia are developing. **Your baby girl's hymen is usually ruptured by the contractions of labor** and remains a thin fold of membrane just inside the vagina. (So much for using the intact hymen as verification of virginity!) As Week 18 ends, the baby weighs about 11 oz (308 g) and measures about 6⅓ inches (160 mm) in length—about the same size as a heavy-duty desktop stapler!

The **baby's movements** are becoming stronger as the ossification process continues and soft cartilage is hardened into bone. Most women feel movement for the first time between Weeks 17 and 20. Mothers who are slim may feel their babies move much earlier than heavier moms will. **Feeling movement helps form the attachment or emotional bond between you and your baby that will last a lifetime.**

Food Facts The **cholesterol** you eat in your diet doesn't have as much influence on your blood-cholesterol level as the fats you eat. Here's how the fat in your diet influences the amount of total and LDL cholesterol in your bloodstream:

1. Unsaturated fats increase levels of good HDL and decrease levels of bad LDL.
2. Saturated fats increase levels of good HDL and increase levels of bad LDL.
3. Trans fats decrease levels of good HDL and increase levels of bad LDL. (Bad all the way around. ☹)

Childbirth in Other Cultures Mayan birth attendants traditionally cheer the mother on with a repetitive chant if she seems to be tiring. Those attending the birth will often talk to the laboring woman to help her relax, to encourage her, and to reassure her.

Chart your waist size and weight here and on page 181.

WAIST SIZE   WEIGHT

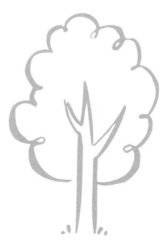

You can learn many things from children. How much patience you have, for instance.

FRANKLIN P. JONES

LMP Week 21

DAY 127	DATE:
	139 days to go

DAY 128	DATE:
	138 days to go

 Over the next three days, your baby's **legs** will approach their final relative proportions. Generally, the baby will be born about 147 days (plus or minus 15 days) from the time the mother first feels her baby move. **Make the calculation** and see how close it comes to the actual day of your baby's birth.

NO MORE ACHING BACK *Suggestion #9:*
Sleep on a **moderately firm mattress** that offers good back support. If your mattress is sagging, you can shore it up somewhat by putting a piece of plywood under it. You may also find that sleeping on the floor makes your back feel great (it's just difficult to know how to situate your bulging tummy).

If your back continues to bother you or the pain worsens, **call your practitioner** before taking any painkiller or drug.

Childbirth in Other Cultures Historically, the tradition among the Dayak people of Borneo was that a medicine man and his assistant visit a woman having a difficult labor. The assistant would stand outside the hut with a moon-colored stone tied to his belly. The medicine man, massaging and soothing the woman, would shout instructions to him to move the stone in imitation of the baby's movements, an act of magical transference.

 The **amniotic fluid is the perfect substance** to support your baby's movement. The baby can move in any way his or her brain and muscles direct: spinning, jackknifing, turning, and somersaulting. The amniotic fluid plays a major role in your baby's growth and development. It keeps him or her buoyant, warm, and clean. It even gives baby something to occasionally swallow so he or she can practice digesting and excreting waste.

The amniotic fluid that surrounds your baby is **completely replaced by your system every three hours.** Drinking plenty of fluids helps support that replacement and keeps your tissues functioning well, too.

Food Facts **Heart-healthy/brain-healthy tips** for monitoring the fat in your diet:

1. Avoid buying foods with unhealthy fat by reading the Nutrition Facts labels.
2. Don't order fast food, fried food, or baked goods unless you know they're trans fat free.
3. Switch from using butter to liquid natural plant oils, especially in cooking.
4. Limit red meat; choose lean cuts of hormone-free grass-fed meats.
5. Get most of your protein from organic beans and peas rather than from meat.
6. Eat low-fat organic dairy foods; limit full-fat cheeses.
7. Eat at least one food source of omega-3 fats daily.

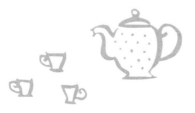

Before I got married, I had six theories about bringing up children; now I have six children and no theories.

JOHN WILMOT, EARL OF ROCHESTER

For Your Health **Fluids are essential** for good health and efficient functioning during pregnancy, since water makes up 55 to 60 percent of your body's weight and 99 percent of the fluid in the amniotic cavity. **Remember to always carry water with you and drink a measured amount between meals.**

DAY 129	DATE:
	137 days to go

Your baby's **legs** now look well proportioned. A newborn's arms and legs appear rather short. That's normal. They'll get longer when your child moves from crawling to walking.

Sleeping position becomes an important consideration during pregnancy. Again, you'll want to try to **sleep on your left side** rather than on your back or your stomach to maximize blood flow.

Did You Know? If you can, fall asleep on your left side, preferably with the left leg straight and the right leg bent and resting on a pillow. This position will relieve pressure on a major vein (the vena cava) which can be restricted by the weight of your uterus. **If you wake up and notice that you're on your stomach or back, don't worry. Just roll over to your left side and try it again.**

Consider This Even though you may be feeling considerably better this trimester, pity the mom who is carrying **twins, triplets, or more**. She may actually be sicker longer because she has higher levels of pregnancy hormones in her system. ☹

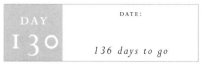

DAY 130	DATE:
	136 days to go

In about a week, lanugo will completely cover your baby's body, although **it will be concentrated around the head, neck, and face.**

Your hair and nails tend to grow rapidly now that you're pregnant because of improved circulation and metabolism caused by pregnancy hormones. If you've ever wanted long, chip-resistant natural nails, now's the time!

For Your Health If you are considering going to a salon or spa for a nail treatment or a change in hair color, **check with your health-care provider first**.

What do you want to be sure to remember?

_____

_____

_____

_____

_____

_____

_____

_____

(See page 102 for more space to write.)

People who say they sleep like a baby usually don't have one.
LEO J. BURKE

DAY **131**	DATE: *135 days to go*	DAY **132**	DATE: *134 days to go*

Your baby's **heart is growing stronger** and stronger. By this time (after Week 18), your baby's heartbeat can be detected by a stethoscope. If your health-care provider forgets to offer, ask if you can listen during your next prenatal visit.

You may notice that **your gums are sensitive and sometimes swell and bleed**. Like other changes, gum sensitivity results from increased levels of pregnancy hormones.

Check with your dentist if you experience severe gum pain or discomfort, or if you are considering any other dental treatments or procedures.

Did You Know? The umbilical cord is so well engineered that the bloodstream travels at four miles an hour and completes the **round-trip through the cord and through the baby in only 30 seconds.**

The baby's arms and legs move with **noticeably more force** now as the muscles strengthen and the bones become stronger. Your baby's sleep habits begin to appear—periods of drowsiness and sleep alternate with periods of activity. Sometimes the mother can detect and anticipate these **sleep cycles.**

You may notice that you're feeling a little **more emotionally stable** and are experiencing fewer mood swings. Some irritability and absentmindedness or forgetfulness are common. After all, you're probably still tired much of the time, especially if you have other children, and you may be distracted by thoughts of the baby.

Did You Know? In a week or two, your baby's sleep patterns will incorporate the rapid eye movements under closed lids **associated with dreaming.** Rather than dreaming, rapid eye movement or REM sleep helps your baby's brain develop.

Childbirth in Other Cultures In the United States, most women lie prone with their shoulders propped up when they give birth. However, **most women in other cultures give birth in vertical positions**: kneeling, sitting, squatting, standing, or even being suspended from ropes or poles. Being upright has the advantage of speeding labor by working with the force of gravity.

> *Chart your waist size and weight here and on page 181.*

WAIST SIZE   WEIGHT

*Nothing has a stronger influence psychologically on their environment,
and especially on their children, than the unlived lives of the parents.*
CARL JUNG

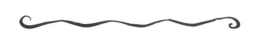

DAY 133	DATE:
	133 days to go

Right now, **your baby looks like a miniature newborn**. Baby's face looks peaceful with closed eyes, nostrils, and a nicely formed mouth. Every once in a while, his or her thumb or finger will slip into the mouth and your baby will practice sucking.

Break out the sparkling apple juice—**today is an important milestone in your pregnancy!** You're now at the halfway point: 19 weeks accomplished, 19 weeks to go. From now on, your body will be preparing to give birth and your baby's systems will develop enough to sustain life outside your uterus.

Did You Know? **Twins** can sometimes be identified by separate heart sounds, especially if their heartbeats differ in rate by more than ten beats a minute. More commonly, ultrasound visualization is used.

Food Facts Vitamins A, D, E, and K are called **"fat-soluble" vitamins** because they bind to the fat in our diet and are stored in abundance in the liver and fatty tissues of the body. Therefore, it takes a long period of deficiency for the body to be depleted of these vitamins, even during pregnancy. However, if these vitamins are oversupplied, they can reach toxic levels.

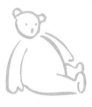

TIME TO REFLECT
What baby names are on the top of your list?

What do you want to be sure to remember?

(See page 102 for more space to write.)

Too often we give children answers to remember rather than problems to solve.
ROGER LEWIN

Week 20 Begins

DAY 134	DATE: 132 days to go

During this week, your baby's brain will begin to grow rapidly. **This rapid brain growth continues until your child is five years old.** In addition, your baby's **lungs** will begin to secrete surfactant—a substance that permits them to inflate and prepare to accept air. Right now, surfactant is only present in small amounts.

The baby may be roused from sleep by external sounds or movements: sudden loud noises, loud music, even the vibrations of a car or washing machine can stir the baby into activity.

By this time in your pregnancy, your practitioner may recommend that **you reduce your level of exertion** at work or even change job duties if your work involves strenuous lifting, bending below your waist, carrying, or climbing ladders or stairs. The idea is to avoid physical stress and strain that could tax your pregnancy.

For Your Information **"Spider veins"** (bright red elevations of the skin radiating from a central body) may develop on your chest, neck, face, back, and legs. If you had them during your first pregnancy, you'll probably have them again. Like other vein changes, these, too, tend to disappear after childbirth.

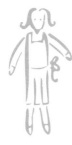

DAY 135	DATE: 131 days to go

By today, your baby's head hair will be visible and the eyebrows are beginning to show. No matter how dark his or her hair will become, **the baby's hair is now completely unpigmented.** In three to four weeks, the eyebrows will look like white streaks; right now, the hair on your baby's head is white and very short.

Your blood was tested for iron sufficiency at your first prenatal appointment; however about 20 percent of women don't retain enough iron as their pregnancy progresses. If you don't have enough iron in your diet, your body doesn't produce as many red blood cells, and fewer red blood cells mean less circulating oxygen in your system. **Women with anemia (iron deficiency) may feel weak, tired, out of breath, and may look pale; on the other hand, you may have no symptoms at all if your anemia is mild.**

Did You Know? **Preventing iron-deficiency anemia is easy.** Eat foods high in iron such as meat, chicken, fish, eggs, dried beans, and fortified grains. Cook with cast-iron pots and pans. Make sure foods high in vitamin C are included daily and get up to 800 mcg in folic acid from your prenatal supplement, orange juice, and dark-green, leafy vegetables.

IMPORTANT: In addition to your prenatal vitamins, your health-care provider may have you take an iron supplement. While the pills are critical to your health, iron is toxic when taken by children. **If you have other children at home, treat iron tablets and your prenatal vitamins as you would any other poison. Store them with great care.**

We call a child's mind "small" simply by habit; perhaps it is larger than ours, for it can take in almost anything without effort.

CHRISTOPHER MORLEY

Childbirth in Other Cultures Umbilical cord cutting is an important ritual in many cultures. Among some tribal cultures in the Philippines, the cord is measured until it touches the baby's forehead and then is cut. The extra length of cord insures that the baby will be "wise."

DAY 136	DATE:
	130 days to go

At this point, your **baby is very lean**. Only about 3.5 percent of his or her body weight is due to fat. This proportion will change in the next weeks and months, as the fat the baby accumulates is a backup source of nourishment and energy.

While dizziness or fainting may be a sign of anemia, it may also indicate that **your blood-sugar level** is low. To keep your blood-sugar level stable, eat small meals every two hours and carry a nutritious snack with you for a quick blood-sugar-level lift.

Did You Know? A blood test is used to diagnose iron-deficiency anemia. Fortunately, while pregnant women may suffer symptoms, unborn babies rarely do. The mother's iron supply is depleted to serve the pregnancy, and it takes about a year to rebuild. Thus, **women who get pregnant before their babies are a year old are more likely than other women to experience iron-deficiency.**

Childbirth in Other Cultures The Punjab of India and the Yahgan of Tierra del Fuego traditionally massage a woman's back and abdomen during labor. Other cultures help her push by applying pressure to her abdomen, squeezing her during contractions, or wrapping her with a belt or a binder during labor.

DAY 137	DATE:
	129 days to go

Sometime during the next three days, **lanugo covers your baby's body.**

You may continue to notice **leg and foot cramps and some mild swelling** of the ankles and feet. Prolonged standing, fatigue, ligaments stretching with your growing uterus, false labor, gas, and constipation may be responsible for cramping. Check in with your health-care provider when you have cramps.

Food Facts **If you don't eat fish**, you can get omega-3 fatty acids from fortified eggs and dairy products, and from organic walnuts, cashews, and pecans. When nuts are rancid, their omega-3s have oxidized and disappeared.

Childbirth in Other Cultures If the midwife attending a birth in the Yucatán Peninsula is concerned about the progress of labor, a common traditional remedy is to give the laboring woman raw egg to swallow. The woman swallows the egg, shudders with revulsion, and regurgitates it. The heaving usually brings on powerful contractions that complete the process of labor.

Chart your waist size and weight here and on page 182.

WAIST SIZE   WEIGHT

Never teach your child to be cunning
for you may be certain that you will be one of the first victims of his shrewdness.
JOSH BILLINGS

DAY	DATE:
1**38**	*128 days to go*

If your baby is a boy, by today the testes will have begun their descent from the pelvis into the scrotum. Remember that ovaries and the testes are formed from the same tissue. The ovaries will remain in place, however. There is another **interesting parallel between male and female systems.** The same tissue that forms the external larger labia in girls comes together and fuses to form the scrotum in boys. The line of that fusion (called the *raphe*) can be seen extending from the base of the penis to the anus and forms during Week 12. It's quite apparent in newborn boys.

While you may be noticing varicose veins in your legs, the veins around your rectum are also susceptible to swelling due to pressure from fluid retention, weight gain, and constipation during pregnancy. These are called **hemorrhoids**, and they may bleed, itch, and cause pain. The best way to prevent hemorrhoids is to avoid becoming constipated.

Consult with your practitioner regarding ways to prevent constipation. Rectal bleeding may also be caused by tears in the anus that occur because of constipation. **Report any rectal bleeding to your practitioner.** A medical diagnosis should be made just in case there might be another cause besides constipation.

Did You Know? You already know that the position of the baby's mouth and anus stabilized the formation of the spinal cord on Day 9. In the early development of the digestive system, the mouth and anus were ultimately connected by the developing esophagus, stomach, large and small intestines, and the rectum.

DAY	DATE:
1**39**	*127 days to go*

Even though his or her eyelids are fused, your baby is now **making blinking movements.** The spine, ribs, and long bones of the arms and legs have **hardened into bone.** The base of the baby's skull is the first to form. At this point, the skull plates that cover the forehead, temples, and top and back of the skull are present and made of cartilage.

Your practitioner may report that your heart rate has increased somewhat during this month. That's normal and just a sign that **your body is having to work a little harder to maintain the pregnancy.**

Food Facts Protein (formed by amino acids) creates cells that become the structure of your baby's body and the placenta. It builds red blood cells, enzymes that break down antibodies (that protect against illness), and hormones for you and your baby. **Women who don't get enough protein risk compromising placental and fetal growth and baby's brain function.**

For Your Information **If you prefer vegetables, pasta, and legumes to meat**, you can fulfill your daily protein requirement during pregnancy by eating dried organic beans, peas, lima beans, natural barley, quinoa, and cooked oat bran/oatmeal, as well as whole-grain bread, uncooked wheat germ, and whole-wheat macaroni and spaghetti.

When you are dealing with a child, keep all your wits about you, and sit on the floor.
AUSTIN O'MALLEY

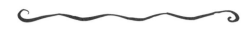

TIME TO REFLECT

Who is your closest friend and supporter?

_____

_____

_____

_____

DAY **140**	DATE: _____ *126 days to go*

The **size and strength** of your baby's hands have improved so that by now, he can grip with some force. **If your baby is a female,** her uterus is completely formed and has just undergone its most rapid period of growth.

At the end of this fifth month of pregnancy, **your uterus has reached your belly button.** The baby in that uterus measures about 7½ inches (191 mm) in length and is about the size of a Barbie or Ken doll. In less than two weeks, the baby has gained more than 3½ oz (100 g). Right now your baby weighs about a pound (about 460 g). Hold a pound package of butter in your hand. That's about how much your baby weighs right now and how heavy baby would feel if you could hold him or her.

Childbirth in Other Cultures Historically, traditional midwives in Sumatra cut the baby's umbilical cord with a flute to make sure the child has a good voice.

Did You Know? After birth, your baby may sneeze and his or her nose may be runny from accumulated amniotic fluid. **If you didn't know this, you might think your baby had already caught a cold.**

For Your Information **The bacteria and viruses that cause infections, colds, and flu are introduced by inhaling germs from an uncovered sneeze or cough, eating or drinking from an infectious person's utensils or cup, or touching one's nose or mouth with unclean hands.** Germs linger in the body by sticking to the nose and mouth cells and the red blood cells. That's why frequent handwashing and avoiding contact with affected people can reduce your chances of getting a cold or the flu.

What do you want to be sure to remember?

_____

_____

_____

_____

_____

_____

_____

_____

_____

_____

_____

(See page 102 for more space to write.)

Respect the child. Be not too much his parent. Trespass not on his solitude.

RALPH WALDO EMERSON

*What do you want to remember about your **Fifth Month**?*

Lunar Month 6

THINGS TO DO THIS MONTH:

* Report any fatigue, weakness, or breathlessness to your health-care provider.

* Keep all vitamins and supplements out of children's reach.

* Maintain your blood-sugar level by eating small meals every two hours.

* Take steps to reduce leg and foot cramps; report uterine or abdominal cramps to your practitioner.

* Maintain a diet high in omega-3 fatty acids.

* Make sure your high-quality protein intake is adequate.

* Continue to dilute concentrated juice.

* Discuss any sexual or sexually transmitted disease concerns with your health-care provider.

* Get sufficient dietary fiber and whole-grain foods.

* Tell your health-care provider *right away* about severe leg pain or tenderness, warmness, swelling, or redness in your legs.

* If you haven't already, begin gathering some of the items you will need after your baby is born.

* Change position to relieve tingling in arms or legs.

* Practice safe food-handling guidelines for shopping, storing, and preparing food.

* Report severe or sudden swelling in hands and face or a severe headache *immediately* to your health-care provider.

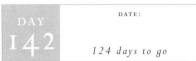

LMP Week 23

DAY 141	DATE:
	125 days to go

The bones of the middle ear **(the three smallest bones in the human body**: the hammer, the anvil, and the stirrup) are beginning to harden to make sound conduction possible. The sound information transmitted to your baby's brain won't trigger an interpretation (e.g., Mommy is speaking, a dog is barking) because your baby has had no experience with the outside world. Only sound intensity seems to register since unexpectedly loud sounds trigger an automatic startle reflex—your baby will blink or "jump" when he or she hears a loud noise.

You can actually touch your own cervix with a clean or gloved hand if you are so inclined. It is a bump toward the end of the upper surface of your vagina. The cervix looks like a doughnut with the dent in the center. Toward the end of the pregnancy it becomes quite difficult to feel on your own due to the changing position of the baby. **You cannot reliably check your own cervical dilation in the third trimester and should not attempt to do so.**

Did You Know? The word **doula** comes from the Greek, meaning "a woman helping another woman." The modern doula is a trained caregiver who provides emotional and physical support to a mother during labor and afterward and helps the dad/partner get involved. A few hospitals have doula programs through which mothers are provided with a doula; otherwise, it's generally a fee-based service.

Childbirth in Other Cultures If an expectant mother in the Ainu tribe of Japan exercises during pregnancy, she is supposed to have a short labor for her reward.

DAY 142	DATE:
	124 days to go

The **baby will gain considerable weight** within the next four weeks. By Week 26, your baby will weigh almost twice as much as he or she does today.

To support the baby's rapid growth, your body needs and stores more protein now than at any other time during your pregnancy.

Food Facts We are **overnourished by fruit juice** because we tend to drink its concentrated form. For example, although we can squeeze ½ cup of juice from one orange, there are actually two oranges in each 8-oz cup of orange juice. Thus, an 8-oz glass of pulp-free orange juice has 120 calories and 0 g of fiber, while a natural orange has half the calories, about 3 g of fiber, and half the fruit sugar.

Consider This When you drink fruit juice, dilute it by half with purified water. Better yet, enjoy the fruit juice in its natural container with the addition of fiber, which helps slow down its absorption in the bowel and **helps you feel full without overeating.**

A B C

If you want a baby, have a new one. Don't baby the old one.
JESSAMYN WEST

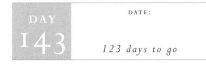

DAY 143	DATE:
	123 days to go

The first movements you feel your baby make will be caused by arm and leg activity. These first motions are called **"quickening."**

Quickening is a notable event for most pregnant women. Excluding ultrasound visualization, **it may mark the first time they feel their baby is "real."**

Childbirth Then and Now Almost all cultures have views on the moment when the spirit, or life force, enters a baby. Before the causes of conception were understood, people thought that babies were put directly into their mothers' wombs. Prior to that time, the children's spirits were thought to reside in natural formations, like rocks, ponds, or trees. Thus, from this perspective, all people were "children of the earth" because that was their first home. The views of Western society have varied. The Catholic Church believes the spirit of the baby enters with conception; English common law (the codes upon which American laws were built) felt that it enters when the mother first feels the baby move. Today, these beliefs are still debated, as people in the twenty-first century **ponder when life begins.**

Food Facts If you happen to be pregnant when fresh fruit is available, strawberries and raspberries are great sources of vitamin C. Three-fourths of a cup of strawberries contains more than half of your day's requirement. Berries should not be washed until you are ready to eat them. They may break apart, and wet berries become moldy much faster.

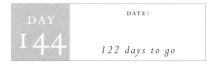

DAY 144	DATE:
	122 days to go

Your baby's respiratory system is still quite immature. Much more development must take place before the lungs can trap and transfer oxygen to the baby's bloodstream and can release carbon dioxide when the baby exhales.

Right now, there's about 350 ml of **amniotic fluid** in your uterus—the equivalent of a cup and a half. As your uterus enlarges, you may notice some aching in your lower abdomen due to the stretching of the muscles and ligaments that support the uterus. The aching may be especially noticeable when you get up from a chair, change position, or get out of bed.

The **pelvic pain** might be sharp, but if it is occasional and not accompanied by any other symptoms, there is probably no cause for alarm.

Food Facts **Protein is filling—it helps satisfy hunger.** Consider these high-protein suggestions: hard-cooked enriched egg; thoroughly cooked barbecued albacore in a lightly dressed salad; cheese on whole-grain macaroni; vegetarian chili; organic black beans on whole-grain rice with salsa . . . YUM!

TIME TO REFLECT
What do you want most for your child?

....
....
....
....
....

I do not believe in a child world. . . . I believe the child should be taught from the very first that the whole world is his world, that adult and child share one world, that all generations are needed.

PEARL S. BUCK

DAY
145

DATE:

121 days to go

DAY
146

DATE:

120 days to go

The heat-producing **brown fat** that the baby has stored in his or her neck, chest, and crotch area will diminish after birth. During months 8 and 9, **white fat** will be deposited under your baby's skin.

As your uterus becomes larger, you may have some concerns about having **sex during pregnancy.** For the most part, let your own sexual comfort be your guide. Certain positions may be more comfortable than others. Also, you may notice changes in your sexual responsiveness: for some women, it's easier to have an orgasm; for others, it's more difficult.

Since sex is part of a normal, loving relationship, sex during pregnancy is encouraged unless you have complications, experience vaginal bleeding or fluid loss, or are having twins or multiple babies. **If you have questions or concerns, check with your practitioner. Be sure to protect yourself from sexually transmitted disease.**

Food Facts If you're feeling **hungry for something sweet and cold**, opt for a no-added-sugar juice bar, sherbet, sorbet, or frozen yogurt instead of ice cream. While superpremium ice cream like Häagen-Dazs, Ben & Jerry's, and Baskin-Robbins can be very satisfying, their ice cream contains huge amounts of saturated fat and calories. For example, there is upwards of 290 cal and 19 g of saturated fat in a single 4-oz serving of Häagen-Dazs Mint Chip ice cream. Four ounces equates to about seven tablespoon-sized bites. **Twenty grams of saturated fat is the recommended daily limit.**

Your baby's body is becoming better proportioned. Although the head still looks large in relation to the body, the legs, arms, and trunk are not as short.

As your skin stretches, **your belly may begin to itch.**

For Your Comfort Since scratching provides no relief, you may want to keep the area moist with lotion and try to prevent excessive weight gain, as it will only add to your discomfort.

Childbirth Then and Now Superstition has always played a role in assisting difficult labor. **According to Pliny the Elder (23–75 CE), the ancient Romans thought people should not cross their legs or clasp their hands near a pregnant woman.** In Europe in the late 1880s, the ringing of church bells was thought to hasten childbirth.

Chart your waist size and weight here and on page 182.

WAIST SIZE   WEIGHT

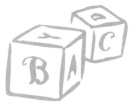

Never help a child with a task at which he feels he can succeed.

MARIA MONTESSORI

DAY 147	DATE: 119 days to go

Fine, downy lanugo covers the baby's entire body, including the head. **During the next six weeks (Weeks 22 through Week 28), the baby will grow in ways that will safeguard his or her survival if born prematurely.** Every day the baby spends growing in the womb is a day filled with developmental progress!

Your **vaginal tissues** become thicker during pregnancy due to increased blood volume.

IMPORTANT: You and your childbirth coach (partner, friend, relative, etc.) should begin taking **childbirth preparation instruction** sometime soon. Such a course will help you understand more about what will happen in the birth process and will help you concentrate on pain control through breathing, relaxation, distraction, and education. If you are giving birth at a hospital, the hospital may have its own course for expectant mothers. Even so, check with other childbirth educators in your area about course availability.

Childbirth Then and Now In colonial America, the pain of labor was thought to be relieved by leaving an axe by the bed with the blade up to "cut the pain," opening the windows, or setting the horses free from the stable. (If only it could be that simple!)

What do you want to be sure to remember?

(See page 120 for more space to write.)

It's a great mistake, I think, to put children off with falsehoods and nonsense, when their growing powers of observation and discrimination excite in them a desire to know about things.

ANNE SULLIVAN

Week 22 Begins

DAY	DATE:
148	*118 days to go*

Your baby's environment is becoming more crowded as he or she is growing and **filling up the space inside the uterus.**

Each day may bring more awareness of the baby's movement. Although the bumps and thumps are now obvious to you, it may be **a few more weeks before someone else can feel the baby move by touching your abdomen.**

For Your Information Studies have indicated that a **doula** can reduce the chance of a cesarean section by 28 percent and reduce the need for pain medication, epidurals, drugs to kick-start labor, and vacuum extractors. A doula-attended birth can also lower the risk of postpartum depression and increase the chances of successful breast-feeding. **The option is WELL worth your consideration.**

Food Facts **Excellent sources of dietary fiber** at 8 g and above include canned vegetarian baked beans, raspberries, boiled artichoke, and cooked green peas, lima beans, black beans, lentils, and split peas. During pregnancy, 28 g of fiber are recommended daily.

Childbirth Then and Now Among the Chagga of Tanzania, there is a saying, "Pay attention to the pregnant woman! There is no one more important than she."

DAY	DATE:
149	*117 days to go*

Throughout this month, changes in the appearance of your baby's skin will take place. Right now, the **skin is wrinkled.** When more fat is deposited and more muscle development takes place, it will begin to look smooth.

Even now, **your breasts are preparing for milk production and nursing.** To produce breast milk of the highest quality, breast-feeding women need to drink 16 cups (up from 13 cups) of water and increase the amount of pregnancy-related nutrients. The exception is iron where the daily value falls by about half. Here are the new daily values for you to switch to:

vitamin A	1,300 µg	vitamin B$_1$	1.7 mg
riboflavin B$_2$	1.6 mg	phosphorus	700 mg
vitamin B$_6$	2 µg	magnesium	320 mg
vitamin B$_{12}$	2.8 µg	vitamin D	200 IU
biotin	35 µg	vitamin K	90 µg
vitamin C	120 mg	molybdenum	50 µg
choline	550 mg	fluoride	3 mg
chromium	45 µg	copper	1,300
vitamin E	19 mg	folic acid	500 to 600 µg
iodine	290 µg	iron	9 to 18 mg
calcium	1,000 mg	manganese	2.6 mg
pantothenic		zinc	12 mg
acid	7mg	niacin	not advised

Source: www.perinatology.com

Food Facts **The value of calcium during pregnancy cannot be overstated.** Monitor your calcium intake carefully—you need 1,000 mg daily. The easiest way to get a quick dose of calcium is to drink a glass of milk.

There are three ways to get something done:
Do it yourself, employ someone, or forbid your children to do it.
MONTE CRANE

Childbirth in Other Cultures Historically, salt and sweet things were forbidden to the Jivaro women of Ecuador when pregnant, in the belief that this deprivation will prevent the fetus from growing too big.

DAY 150	DATE:
	116 days to go

The **baby's skin is not only wrinkled but is also transparent** because it's so thin. Thus, at this time, if you could see your baby, the bones, organs, and blood vessels would be visible, as they lie just beneath the skin.

Leg cramps can be prevented by making dietary changes (adding calcium, reducing phosphorus), sitting with feet elevated rather than standing, and wearing support stockings or leggings. If you do experience a cramp in your calf muscle, stand in a lunge position facing a wall. (The uncramped leg should be in the lead by 2 to 3 feet. Place your hands on the wall for support.) Press the heel of your back leg (the one that's cramped) slowly to the floor. You should feel your muscle begin to stretch out, and the cramp should disappear. Remember not to bounce—you want a slow stretch. Bouncing might cause injury.

Talk to your health-care provider if you have severe leg pain often or you've noticed tender places, warmth, swelling, or redness in your legs.

For Your Health **Iodine is one of the few nutrients regarded as essential.** The thyroid gland uses it to produce a hormone (thyroxine) that controls the way the body's cells use oxygen and release energy. The most common source of iodine is iodized salt. If you are looking for an alternative source, sea

vegetables (kelp)—like sushi *nori*, for example—are a rich source of iodine and other nutrients. The recommended daily value of iodine is 220 mcg.

Childbirth Then and Now According to Thomas Raynalde in *The Byrthe of Mankynde* (1540), "The thynges which helpe the byrthe and make it more easie, are these. First, the woman that laboureth must eyther sytte grovelyng or els upright, leaning backwards, according as it shal seeme commodius and necessary to the partie, or as she is accustomed."

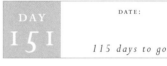

Chart your waist size and weight here and on page 182.

WAIST SIZE   WEIGHT

DAY 151	DATE:
	115 days to go

Your baby continues to grow at a steady pace. More than 6 oz (168 g) of weight—equivalent to a half can of soda—will be gained during this week alone. This **growth spurt** helps your baby prepare for life without the umbilical lifeline.

Like last month, you may notice **aching in the small of your back.**

For Your Health **Take steps to prevent backache.** Lying down, having a massage, and heating the area may soothe aching muscles.

For Your Information **Some urinary tract infections can occur without symptoms.** Your practitioner can test you for the presence of this infection and treat you if you have it.

Fear less, hope more; eat less, chew more; whine less, breathe more; hate less, love more, and all good things are yours.

SWEDISH PROVERB

Did You Know? **Breast milk is 87 percent water, but the remaining 13 percent is the best naturally sustainable food on the planet!**

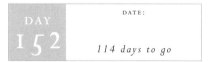

DATE:

DAY
1 5 2

114 days to go

Your baby weighs just under a pound-and-a-half, the equivalent of three 8-oz cups of water. Most of the weight gained during this time in your baby's development is muscle and bone mass and weight increases from growing organs and tissues. Very little fat is being manufactured right now. Ultimately, most of the muscles involved in movement develop before birth, and all those that remain are formed by baby's first birthday. Muscles increase in length and width in order to grow with the skeleton. Their ultimate size depends on how much exercise baby gives them.

As your baby grows, so do you. On average, **expect to gain about a pound a week during this month.**

Did You Know? The **first true bonelike formation** occurs in the baby's breastbone as it joins with the ribs.

Parenting Tip Eco-friendly premoistened baby wipes are useful for cleaning, but they can't disinfect. Environmentally friendly antibacterial surface wipes can help sanitize in restaurants, playgrounds, grocery carts, public transportation, and so on. Use each wipe only once to avoid spreading germs from one surface to another, and dispose of them responsibly.

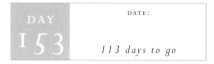

DATE:

DAY
1 5 3

113 days to go

Internal sounds that are heard daily by your baby include the beating of your heart, the sound of your voice resonating as you speak, the sound of air filling your lungs and being exhaled, and the growling noises made by your stomach and intestines.

As the baby's heartbeat becomes louder, it may be possible to hear the baby's heart by placing an ear to your abdomen—a yogalike pose that may be quite impossible for you to achieve, but easy for others! **A stethoscope will help you hear your baby's heart beating loud and strong.**

Did You Know? **Taste buds are formed in abundance** on your baby's tongue and inside its cheeks, some of which will slough off after birth. On average, the tongue will have about 10,000 taste buds that are replaced every two weeks or so.

Childbirth in Other Cultures The custom among most Native American women in the past was to deliver babies in an isolated setting, often along the banks of a stream. A Sioux woman would sit with her legs crossed at the ankle and her thighs separated. Her arms were crossed over her chest, her head was bowed, and her body was bent forward, especially during contractions. It's interesting to note that ancient Egyptian drawings show women in this same cross-legged position, seemingly in the act of giving birth.

Remember, when they have a tantrum, don't have one of your own.
DR. JUDITH KURIANSKY

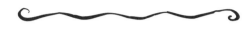

TIME TO REFLECT

Whose facial features do you want your baby to inherit?

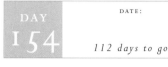

Between now and the baby's due date, his or her feet will almost double in size, from about 1.8 inches (45 mm) to 3.3 inches (83 cm).

Today marks the completion of 22 weeks of pregnancy. At this point, **being pregnant is nothing new—it's become a way of life!** If you are still experiencing some stomach upset and nausea, eating an easily digested snack every two hours may help you feel less nauseous.

Your health may decline if vomiting connected with morning sickness persists throughout the day. **Notify your practitioner that same day if you vomit more than two or three times or you begin vomiting when you haven't before.** In about 5 percent of pregnancies, nausea persists until childbirth. With any luck, that won't include you.

Parenting Tip After having a baby, someone who was with you during delivery should talk to your partner and other children if you were separated from them. Young children, especially, may be worried about your health and well-being. They will need emotional reassurance and will probably have a lot of pressing questions. After you go home, expect immature, babylike behavior from older children—a common, though temporary, response to the birth of a new sibling. It's often a signal that **a child needs extra loving attention.**

What do you want to be sure to remember?

(See page 120 for more space to write.)

Every man is to be envied who is fortunate with his children.

EURIPIDES

LMP Week 25

DAY 155	DATE:
	111 days to go

The smallest blood vessels of the body—the capillaries—are beginning to develop under the baby's skin. As blood fills these new vessels, **they give your baby's skin a red or pinkish appearance,** because the blood in the capillaries is visible.

You may notice **tingling sensations** in your hands and feet from time to time. These symptoms are common and often due to swelling in the wrists and ankles, which puts pressure on the nerves that pass through those narrow spaces. Changing position may bring some relief.

For Your Health Food-borne illness is caused by eating food that contains harmful bacteria, toxins, parasites, viruses, or chemical contaminants. **Eating even a small portion of unsafe food can make you and your baby sick and can interrupt your pregnancy.** Symptoms may appear within hours or weeks of eating a contaminated food.

If you think you have become ill from eating contaminated food, **consult your practitioner.**

Childbirth in Other Cultures According to tradition, when the Taureg women of the Sahara go into labor, they walk up and down the small, sandy hills of their region, returning to their hut when it's time to deliver their babies.

DAY 156	DATE:
	110 days to go

Your baby continues to perform reflex movements that are essential to his or her survival after birth. **Lips and mouth are sensitive,** so if the baby's hand floats near the mouth, he or she may suck the thumb or fingers.

The startle reflex, also present for some time now, rouses baby's body to prepare to protect itself from the unexpected. For example, you may have felt your baby "jump" when he or she hears a loud sound.

For Your Health Prevent food-borne illness by separating raw, cooked, and ready-to-eat foods while shopping, storing, or preparing foods. This practice **prevents cross-contamination.** Store raw meat, poultry, fish, and shellfish in containers in the refrigerator so that the juices don't drip onto other foods.

Childbirth in Other Cultures After giving birth, a Tarong woman of the Philippines is traditionally given a tea made from her charred placenta and a root that is eaten to eliminate "bad air." She is also given a cigar to smoke!

Food Facts **Protect your baby from illness by building up your own immune system.** Protein and vitamin B_5 (pantothenic acid) play a key role in helping your body make antibodies to fight off bacteria and viruses. Even a 25 percent reduction in protein can make a significant difference. And insufficient vitamin B_1 (thiamin) and B_2 (riboflavin) can make normal antibodies less responsive. Fortified eggs are a high-quality source of protein. Cauliflower

It is better to bind your children to you by a feeling of respect, and by gentleness, than by fear.

PUBLIUS TERENTIUS AFER

and crimini mushrooms contain generous amounts of B_5, and romaine lettuce is a rich source of vitamins B_1 and B_2.

DAY 157

DATE:

109 days to go

Right now, your baby's **grip is far more powerful than that of a newborn.**

Mild swelling in your ankles and feet is common and expected.

Contact your practitioner if you have severe or sudden swelling, especially in your hands or around your eyes. Other signs that may accompany swelling, like severe headache, dizziness, or blurred vision, need to be reported *right away.*

For Your Health Prevent the possibility of food poisoning by **avoiding raw and undercooked foods.** Do not eat raw or undercooked beef, poultry, fish, shellfish, ground meat, sushi, or sprouts. Cooked sushi like California Rolls are safe, but seared meats are not. Don't eat raw or partially cooked eggs or foods containing raw eggs; the yolk should be firm.

Consider This **Clean surfaces** protect against germs. Wash your countertops, cutting boards, and hands frequently with warm water and mild natural soap.

Chart your waist size and weight here and on page 182.

WAIST SIZE   WEIGHT

DAY 158

DATE:

108 days to go

Gradually, your **baby's fingernails and toenails lengthen.** They are growing from the nail beds and are beginning to cover the skin itself.

Continue to **prevent urinary tract infections** by drinking plenty of fluids (water and unsweetened organic juices high in vitamin C), avoiding caffeine-containing drinks, thoroughly emptying your bladder when you urinate, minimizing stress, and practicing good hygiene (shower daily and wash your vaginal area gently but thoroughly).

Parenting Tip You won't be giving your baby a full bath until the umbilical cord falls off. **It takes a week or two for the stump of the umbilical cord to dry up and drop off, leaving the healed scar we call the navel.** Even then, remember that, until baby starts crawling, only its bottom, face, and neck will get dirty. First babies probably get bathed more than later-born children because parents have more time than they do with two or more children. A day without a bath is not a disgrace, since the dirty spots can be wiped clean. On the other hand, a bath can be relaxing for both of you.

Don't demand respect as a parent. Demand civility and insist on honesty.
But respect is something you must earn—with kids as well as with adults.
WILLIAM ATTWOOD

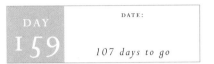

DAY 159

DATE:

107 days to go

Over the next three days, blood vessels will develop in your **baby's lungs.**

If you have hemorrhoids, you may experience some **rectal bleeding** in addition to the usual symptoms of pain and itching.

Did You Know? **Prevention is still the key for treating hemorrhoids:** drink plenty of fluids, eat fresh fruits and vegetables in quantity, avoid sitting in place for hours at a time, exercise moderately, and walk to reduce or minimize their development.

For Your Health Prevent the possibility of food-borne illness by **avoiding unpasteurized** eggs, juice, milk, and milk products made from unpasteurized milk, such as certain cheeses. Substitute fresh, natural juice, eggs, and pasteurized milk in recipes calling for those ingredients. Avoid soft cheeses unless they are made with pasteurized milk.

Parenting Tip If you're ever in a situation where you have to give **a refrigerator-cold bottle** to a hungry baby, don't worry. It's not harmful in any way. The baby can digest cold formula just as well as warm formula; it's just not as appealing.

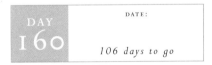

DAY 160

DATE:

106 days to go

The baby's nostrils (which until now have been plugged) begin to open. By today, blood vessels will have developed in the lungs. After birth, **these vessels will allow blood to flow through the lungs to intercept oxygen and circulate it to your baby's tissues.**

For great hygiene, the amniotic fluid that surrounds the baby is removed and replaced by your system **every three hours**. Right now the total daily exchange is equivalent to 6 gal (25.6 l) in volume.

Did You Know? Ultimately, baby will have five kinds of **taste buds** on his or her tongue. The conventional tastes include salty, sour, bitter, and sweet. In addition, **umami**, a savory taste, is the fifth basic taste and at its most delicious seems to be a form of ideal saltiness. Tomatoes and soy sauce are rich in umami components.

For Your Health Outside the home, **freshly prepared fruit juice** that is safer to drink comes from fruit that is washed and juiced immediately before you drink it (like fresh-squeezed orange juice). If you juice your own fruit, wash the fruit thoroughly with soap and water first. Except for lettuce, wash produce in the same way; use a brush to remove surface dirt, if necessary.

Childbirth in Other Cultures For Mayan women in the Yucatán Peninsula, some pain is an expected part of birth, as it is an accepted part of life in general. Traditionally, no attempt is made to protect the pregnant woman by withholding information about labor and childbirth. Pain appears in the stories women tell about their own birth experiences. The storyteller makes it clear that the laboring woman's distress is normal and that her suffering will pass, just as it did for other women.

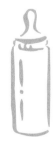

The most important thing a father can do for his children is to love their mother.
THEODORE HESBURGH

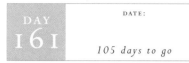

DAY 161

DATE:

105 days to go

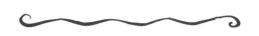

During this month, the **buds for your baby's permanent teeth** will come in high in the gums behind the buds for the baby teeth. The baby's **spine** will ultimately be made up of 33 rings, 150 joints, and 1,000 ligaments, all of which are used to support their body weight. All of those structures will begin to form during this month.

Upward of 50 percent of all pregnant women develop hemorrhoids—painful, swollen veins in the rectum and anus—and may experience some rectal bleeding. **While rectal bleeding does not signal a problem with the baby, it should be reported to your practitioner for evaluation.**

For Your Health Prevent the possibility of food-borne illness by cooking foods properly. Proper cooking makes most foods safe. The best way to tell if a meat, poultry, or egg dish is **cooked to a safe temperature** is to use an inexpensive food thermometer, available at most stores. Reheat soups, sauces, marinades, and gravy to a boil. Reheat leftovers thoroughly and to at least 165°F (74°C), since harmful bacteria can grow between 41°F (5°C) and 139°F (59°C). Foods left out for more than one or two hours, or stored in the refrigerator past three or four days, may contain a toxin that can't be destroyed by cooking. **When in doubt, throw it out!**

Childbirth in Other Cultures The home was and is the primary place of birth among tribal peoples of the world. The second most common place was the birthing hut, a place designated for birth alone or shared with menstruating women. Among modern Western nations, **the Dutch have one of the highest percentages of home births in the world.** One-third of all their babies are born at home.

TIME TO REFLECT
Are there any names to which you would say "Absolutely not!"?

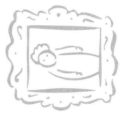

What do you want to be sure to remember?

(See page 120 for more space to write.)

Let your children go if you want to keep them.
MALCOLM FORBES

LMP Week 26

DAY 162	DATE:
	104 days to go

DAY 163	DATE:
	103 days to go

Now that the nostrils have begun to open, your baby will make periodic muscular breathing movements as its body prepares to draw air into the lungs at birth. **These breathing movements stimulate lung development and can be detected by ultrasound.**

At this point in your pregnancy, you may have to adjust your schedule so you **get sufficient rest.**

Did You Know? From Week 15 through Week 28, the **amniotic fluid volume increases** at an average rate of ¼ cup minus 2 teaspoons (50 ml) per week, twice the weekly fluid increase during the first 15 weeks of pregnancy.

Ready to Breast-Feed Breast milk from donors is stored in **human-milk banks.** Sick and premature babies who are prescribed donor milk to supplement their mothers' milk develop far fewer complications than the sick and premature babies who don't receive the supplements. At the time of this writing, the need for donated milk is higher than the supply.

Did You Know? As of this writing, Brazil has the largest number of **human-milk banks** of any country in the world.

Within the next two days, **air sacs** (alveoli) will begin to develop in the baby's lungs. Alveoli continue to form for about nine more years. **Breathing is usually possible by the end of Week 24** because some of the alveoli have developed at the ends of the bronchial tubes and the lung tissue is well supplied with blood. In addition, the membrane that separates the air sacs from the capillaries is thin enough to allow oxygen–carbon dioxide exchange.

By keeping your fat intake low, you will **gain what weight you need to sustain your pregnancy without padding your body with fat.** Avoid high-calorie salad dressing, sauces and gravies, and rich desserts.

Did You Know? **Animal fat** (from beef, chicken, etc.) also contains vitamins A and D. Even so, fat should be eaten sparingly.

For Your Health Prevent the possibility of food-borne illness by **replacing worn cutting boards** once they develop hard-to-clean grooves.

Ready to Breast-Feed There are some people (and nations) who feel so strongly about promoting breast-feeding that they maintain that formula is artificial food and that mothers are **abusing and neglecting their babies by not breast-feeding.** Interesting, huh?

By the time the youngest children have learned to keep the house tidy, the oldest grandchildren are on hand to tear it to pieces.

CHRISTOPHER MORLEY

DAY 164

DATE:

102 days to go

Your baby's lungs are secreting surfactant, a substance that **keeps the lung tissue from sticking to itself and allows the air sacs to inflate.**

Pregnant or not, women need to monitor their **sun exposure** carefully. Any changes you are experiencing in your skin's pigmentation (especially blotchiness) will be darkened by sun exposure, and pregnant skin is especially susceptible to sunburn. An effective DHA-free sunscreen, a wide-brimmed hat, and light-colored long-sleeved cotton clothing offer you the best protection. Again, check with your health-care provider before you do any sunless tanning.

For Your Health **Tanning beds are a concern during pregnancy** not so much because of the UVA and UVB rays emitted by the bulbs (they don't seem to penetrate far enough to harm the baby), but because of the potential for dehydration due to fluid loss and overheating by raising body temperature. Err on the side of safety and avoid them.

Childbirth Then and Now In rural America during the eighteenth century, the birth attendant was paid with whatever the family could afford—chickens, a twist of tobacco, or day work. Sometimes in lieu of payment, a girl child would bear the attendant's name.

Parenting Tip Invest in a baby glider or a rocker. Wood, metal, and upholstered styles are available. **Rocking can soothe a baby, and it will relax you, too.**

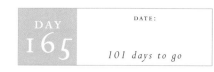

Chart your waist size and weight here and on page 182.

WAIST SIZE   WEIGHT

DAY 165

DATE:

101 days to go

Over the next four days, brain wave activity will begin for your baby's visual and auditory systems. **The senses are developing the kind of connections with the brain that will be useful for interpreting what baby sees and hears after birth.** While the presence of brain wave activity indicates that your baby's eyes have encountered a light source or that your baby's ears have received a sound message, no comprehension is possible yet. This system needs training and practice just like all the others to make any sense of what is seen and heard.

Take it slow and easy when you exercise. The "no pain, no gain" philosophy doesn't work with pregnancy. Concentrate on stretching, balance, working on core strength, and toning. **Continue to avoid bouncing and overly strenuous workouts with implications for dehydration and overheating.**

Be sure your exercises are designed for pregnant women and suitable to your pregnancy. **Check with your practitioner before beginning any program of exercise.**

For Your Health **When eating out,** prevent the possibility of food-borne illness by ordering foods thoroughly cooked and making sure they are served piping hot.

Home is not where you live but where they understand you.
CHRISTIAN MORGENSTERN

Ready to Breast-Feed **You'll want to buy or borrow a breast pump.** The pump helps relieve engorged breasts, and gives your baby the benefits of breastmilk if you are concerned about nursing in public. The pump helps you transfer breastmilk to bottles so others can feed the baby, keeps your milk production up, gives your nipples a break if they are sore, and can be used anywhere. There are adapters for use in your car, but not while driving. ☺ There are many styles of pumps in a range of prices. The Affordable Care Act (ACA) now requires health plans to cover breast-feeding support and supplies, so give your insurance company a call to find out which pumps they cover. You'll want one that's reliable, easy to use, easy to keep clean, and easy to pack up and use away from home.

different cultures. Traditionally, a well-to-do Goajiro Indian woman of Colombia will rest in bed for a month after delivering her first baby. However, among the Yahgan of Tierra del Fuego, a new mother is back gathering shellfish with her tribe less than a day after giving birth.

Parenting Tip Help your new baby follow **a predictable routine.** Once established, your baby's routine, like that of the other family members, should be respected. For example, it's disruptive to wake the baby up from a scheduled (and needed) nap just because a friend or relative is visiting and wants to see the baby. It's nice for people to be interested in the newborn, but it's easier for adults to wait until the baby is ready to see them than for the baby to have to conform to the social needs of adults.

| DAY 166 | DATE:

100 days to go |

By this time, **eyebrows and eyelashes** are usually present. Over the next couple of days, your **baby's fingernails will become noticeable.** While the baby's nails are growing, yours may be growing well, too. **Strong, long, healthy nails often accompany pregnancy** because of improvements in circulation and metabolism.

For Your Health Prevent the possibility of food poisoning. **Place perishable foods in your shopping cart last** and take them straight home after buying them. **Refrigerate perishable foods as soon as possible**, but clearly within one hour if the outside temperature is 90°F (32°C) or above. Your refrigerator should cool to 37°F (3°C) and freeze to 0°F (−18°C).

Childbirth in Other Cultures The amount of recuperation time after childbirth varies considerably among

What do you want to be sure to remember?

(See page 120 for more space to write.)

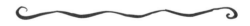

TIME TO REFLECT
Is there anything that you can (or should) do without right now?

A good heart is better than all the heads in the world.
EDWARD BULWER-LYTTON

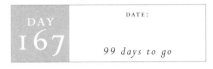

DAY 167

DATE:

99 days to go

Your baby is still lean at 820 g, or almost 2 lb. Its skin is wrinkled and pink to bright red because blood is visible in the tiny blood vessels called capillaries.

For the sake of your circulation, remember to change position frequently. Optimal circulation to the placenta and fetus is possible when you lie on your left side. Walking also aids circulation.

For Your Comfort Avoid standing in a fixed position, if at all possible. If you do stand, do so briefly. Sit with feet elevated.

Ready to Breast-Feed Check to see if a hospital, birthing center, or clinic in your area offers a class on **first-time breast-feeding.** Taking a course like that or locating online resources can also put you in touch with other nursing moms.

Parenting Tip Don't worry if you don't feel overwhelming love for your baby from the moment of birth. Early feelings for a baby can be remarkably ambivalent sometimes. **Enjoy getting to know one another and develop a close and lasting parent-child bond by noting all the beautiful, remarkable, and amazing things about your own little one.**

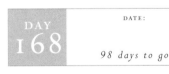

DAY 168

DATE:

98 days to go

This was an important month in your baby's life—the end of the second trimester. In the next three months, **the baby will increasingly be able to survive without the protection of your womb.** At this point, your baby measures at least 9 inches long (230 mm) and weighs at least 1¾ lbs (794 g).

It's important to monitor your blood pressure during pregnancy for signs of elevation. **Unsafe blood pressure changes are most common after this week**, when the proportion of red blood cells to plasma increases and the "relaxation effect" that the hormone progesterone has on the blood vessels reaches its peak.

IMPORTANT: When your blood pressure is high, your heart and other organs have to work harder to circulate blood through vessels that have narrowed. **High blood pressure can limit blood flow to your baby and reduce the amount of food and oxygen available to it.**

For Your Health **Prevent the possibility of foodborne illness** by thawing frozen meats, poultry, fish, and shellfish in the refrigerator, microwave, or in cold water changed every 30 minutes (this keeps the surface chilled). Cook foods immediately after thawing.

Ready to Breast-feed Early on, a breast-fed baby will be hungry about every two hours or so. Baby's automatic reflexes help it find the food source by smell and turn toward it when his or her cheek is stroked. **Latching on** is the process of getting your baby to take enough of your nipple and areola into its mouth to effectively suck out the milk. Get comfortable so your milk will flow. Help the baby latch on by cupping your breast into a *U* so your fingers are parallel to your baby's lips and gently squeeze down so the baby can take the right "bite" and latch on. If the connection is a good one, you can see your baby's jaw move and hear the milk being swallowed and the baby breathing out after he or she swallows.

Hugs can do great amounts of good—especially for children.
PRINCESS DIANA

*What do you want to remember about your **Sixth Month**?*

Lunar Month 7

THINGS TO DO THIS MONTH:

* Count kicks (hiccups don't count); there should be ten or more in a two-hour period.

* Take lots of breaks during the day to rest, since you may be short of breath as your baby grows larger.

* Expect your sleep to be interrupted by the baby's movements.

* Get to know a lactation consultant in your area.

* Purchase a car safety seat.

* Avoid foods that cause discomfort.

* Eat foods with probiotics to reduce the risk of yeast infections.

* Get back to your program of exercise/walking.

* Discuss any plans for air travel with your health-care provider.

* Contact your health-care provider *immediately* if you have a severe headache, blurry vision, sudden weight gain, dizziness, or swelling of the hands and face.

LMP Week 27

DAY 169	DATE:
	97 days to go

DAY 170	DATE:
	96 days to go

Today is a very significant day: Your baby's lungs are now capable of breathing air! By the end of this week, your baby will grow about ½ inch (12.7 mm) longer—that much more prepared for life outside your womb. **Baby's goal weight is at least 1,000 g, or about 2 lb.**

Now that your baby can breathe air, you can breathe a sigh of relief! With sufficient air sacs and surfactant, **your baby will have a much easier time breathing by itself and adapting to the outside world.**

Childbirth Then and Now Many women kneel during labor, resting their upper bodies on a chair, tree stump, or their own arms and elbows. This labor position was referred to in the Bible and by Roman poets, was used in Germany during the Middle Ages, and was popular among Native North American tribal women.

Parenting Tip **Parents are often concerned that their babies will get too cold or too hot when they sleep.** You can test to see if your baby is cozy by touching the back of his or her neck. (Be sure your hand is not cold by running your hands under warm water first.) If the baby's neck is warm and dry, he or she is at a comfortable temperature. If the back of its neck is damp, baby may be too hot. If the neck is cool, you might want to add a blanket. Don't use the temperature of the baby's hands or feet as a guide. They are usually cool no matter what the temperature of the rest of the baby's body.

If your baby is a boy, sometime within the next three months, his testes will have completely descended. **Passage of the boy's testes into his scrotum** may be prompted by the increased pressure in the abdomen due to the development of the intestines.

If you have diabetes, your baby will begin to put on more weight than normal from this point on. With diabetes, either the pancreas doesn't produce as much insulin as needed in the body to break down sugars for energy, or the body is unresponsive to the insulin produced. Some women begin their pregnancies with diabetes; other women develop gestational diabetes **because** of pregnancy. Gestational diabetes generally clears up after the baby is born.

Food Facts **Diabetic or not, 30 mcg of chromium and 2 mg of manganese daily support glucose regulation in the pancreas.** Good dietary sources of chromium are oysters and natural beef, eggs, chicken, wheat germ, green peppers, apples, bananas, and spinach. Food sources of manganese include healthy cooked brown rice, garbanzo beans, boiled spinach, whole-grain rye, cooked tempeh, and cooked soybeans.

Chart your waist size and weight here and on page 182.

WAIST SIZE

WEIGHT

A child is a curly, dimpled lunatic.

RALPH WALDO EMERSON

Childbirth in Other Cultures The Bukidnon of Mindanao in the Philippines consider the placenta to be "the brother" of the baby. By tradition, they bury the placenta under the house and believe that the spirit of the placenta returns to the sky.

Parenting Tip **Babies will stop nursing or bottle-feeding when they are full.** Don't start urging bottle-fed babies to finish the bottle or you will risk training them to overeat. A newborn's stomach is only about the size of his or her little fist, so your baby will need to feed often and in relatively small amounts at first.

Did You Know? It generally **takes the milk-producing cells of the breasts about two hours to manufacture enough milk for the next feeding.** That timing is usually perfect, as the baby can digest one feeding in about two hours before waking up hungry again!

DAY 171	DATE:
	95 days to go

Thankfully, your baby's **lungs** continue their rapid growth.

You will still need about an extra 300 calories per day now, as you enter the last three months of your pregnancy. Altogether, it takes about 77,100 calories to build a baby. (Fortunately, not all at once!)

Ready to Breast-Feed **It's never too early to talk to other mothers about their breast-feeding experiences.** The Internet offers exceptional opportunities to ask questions, get advice, and join moms' groups in order to connect with other women in your area who are learning to breast-feed and dealing with the same issues you are.

Parenting Tip Hold your baby to your shoulder to **burp him or her after a feeding** or try laying baby on your lap, tummy down with his or her head turned a little to the side. Rub baby's back from the bottom up or pat gently. You can also burp a baby by sitting him or her on your lap, placing a hand on baby's chest, and leaning him or her forward while gently patting his or her back. Swallowed air is uncomfortable.

TIME TO REFLECT
This week marks the beginning of your third—and last—trimester of pregnancy. As you look back on your baby's growth and your pregnancy experience so far, what are some of the moments you remember best?

DAY 172	DATE:
	94 days to go

Your baby's brain continues its rapid growth! Do everything you know to do to energize that brain!

You may notice some vaginal itching periodically. Vaginal itching may be due to a yeast infection or lack of regular hygiene (regular cleansing with mild, nondrying soap and water or with unscented mineral oil). It is also one of the symptoms associated with gestational diabetes. **Let your practitioner know if you feel itchy.**

There are times when parenthood seems nothing but feeding the mouth that bites you.
PETER DE VRIES

Food Facts Fermented foods like kimchi, natural yogurt, and kefir contain probiotics that many consider superfoods. **Probiotics** are some 400 species of live "friendly bacteria" that are naturally present in the digestive tract and vagina. Probiotics keep the balance between healthy and harmful bacteria in your system in check and help produce vitamin K. There are many delicious forms of kimchi and beneficial yogurt and kefir to try if you don't think you're a fan.

For Your Health There are naturally low-sugar, low-fat, and nonfat versions of **yogurt**. Avoid brands that add fat. Check the levels of active live cultures in the yogurt—the more live cultures there are, the more health benefits you can receive. Plain yogurt can be substituted for milk in many recipes. Some women who are lactose intolerant can tolerate organic yogurt.

Ready to Breast-Feed **Pillows and other soft supports are a nursing mother's best friends.** Have several pillows available so that you can experiment with the most comfortable arrangement for the two of you that puts your baby at just the right level for comfortable and effective nursing. Solicit advice from other moms, your health-care provider, and lactation consultants. Consider using a travel pillow for your neck. It will help you be more comfortable no matter where you feed the baby, especially during the middle of the night!

Parenting Tip You might find that placing the baby on a pillow or soft support on your lap allows you to rest your nursing arm on a pillow while the baby is feeding. If you nurse in bed, you may want several pillows to rest on or a bed pillow with arms for comfort.

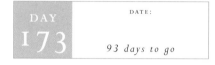

By this time, your **baby's brain wave patterns are similar to those of a full-term baby at birth.** Activity is beginning in the portions of the brain that process visual and auditory information.

Driving a vehicle may be continued until your size makes you uncomfortable or restricts your movement. The shoulder strap shouldn't be uncomfortable. Push the lap belt under your tummy. Until that time, take all the same safety precautions you would at any other time: **1.** Wear your seat belt every time you drive, never drive while "in a hurry" or when you're distracted. **2.** Stay within the speed limits. **3.** Drive defensively, watching out for other motorists.

Consider This As your family gets larger, it may become more and more of a challenge for you and your partner to get time to yourselves not just for intimacy but for doing all the things that make you feel connected and comfortable with each other. Plan regular time together, even if it's just a half-hour walk while a reliable adult watches the baby. And plan to start dating your partner again so you'll have an opportunity to look forward to going out.

Parenting Tip **When you feed your baby, hold him or her in one arm for one feeding and in the other arm for the next** so the baby can practice looking to the left and to the right and you can enjoy him or her from a different perspective. **Study your child, stroke the skin, hold their hand, smile, and stare deeply into their eyes. Love begins here.**

Who knows the thoughts of a child?

NORA PERRY

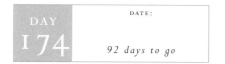

DAY 174 DATE:

92 days to go

During this month, the forebrain or the portion of the baby's brain just behind the forehead will enlarge to cover all other developed brain structures, while still maintaining its hemisphere divisions. **As a result, some significant brain developments will occur.**

As your baby grows physically stronger, his or her thumping and bumping will become stronger, too. You can monitor your baby's movement by **counting his or her kicks**, rolls, stretches, or pushes. (Hiccuping doesn't count.) At least 10 kicks should be felt within a two-hour period. The best time to monitor movements is when your baby is most active; the best position for you to be in is sitting up or lying on your left side (not on your back).

Let your practitioner know if your baby kicks fewer than 10 times in two consecutive hours.

Parenting Tip If you're bottle-feeding, **shake the formula in the bottle to distribute the warmed milk evenly.** Test the temperature of the bottled milk by squirting a drop or two on the inside of your wrist. If the milk feels comfortably warm, it's the right temperature for the baby.

IMPORTANT: Chloride is an element that combines with **sodium** to allow fluids to move freely within cells, maintains the stomach's acidity, and is the most common component of spinal fluid. As an element, chlorine is added to public drinking water to help eliminate diseases like typhoid fever found in contaminated water. Bottled water isn't necessarily cleaner or safer to drink. The CDC maintains that optimal fluoride concentrations in drinking water **reduce tooth decay in children and adults by 25 percent.** Most Americans receive sufficient

chloride through their drinking water and as sodium chloride in table salt. Check with your practitioner about fluoride levels in your water and what they might mean for your developing baby.

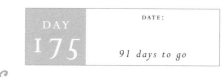

DAY 175 DATE:

91 days to go

Your baby has grown ½ inch (13 mm) in just seven days! **Sounds like adolescence, doesn't it?**

As your baby gets bigger, **you may notice some shortness of breath.** As your growing baby presses on your diaphragm—the tissue that divides your lungs from your intestines—it becomes harder to fill your lungs completely and to breathe out all the air.

IMPORTANT: To help manage any **breathlessness**, slow down, minimize stress, get sufficient rest, and reduce your activity level.

For Your Information About **95 percent of your baby's alveoli**, or respiratory air sacs, develop after birth. About 50 million alveoli (one-sixth of the adult number) are present in the lungs of a full-term newborn. The adult complement of alveoli will be present by age eight.

Ready to Breast-Feed **A board-certified lactation consultant is a professional who trains women to breast-feed.** Lactation consultants meet with new mothers soon after they've given birth to answer questions and demonstrate technique. Some are also private practitioners who can help women at home. Get to know a lactation consultant before you give birth so that you're familiar with the process of breast-feeding before you've got a hungry baby in your arms. Your practitioner and experienced moms can steer you in the right direction.

Better to be driven out from among men than to be disliked of children.
R. H. DANA

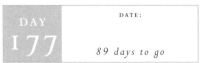

LMP Week 28

DAY 176	DATE:
	90 days to go

Baby's hands can grip with such strength that they will be fisted at birth.

As your growing baby becomes more and more active, you may notice that **your sleep is sometimes interrupted** by his or her restlessness.

Consider This You might want a **representational keepsake of your pregnancy** in the form of artistic photographs or having your belly cast in plaster and painted, decorated, or even bronzed. This remembrance can help you reflect on what it meant to be pregnant, how big you actually got, and how fleeting those moments are in life.

Childbirth in Other Cultures Traditionally, the Pawnee women of North America and women of West Micronesia squat during labor, resting their backs against the back of a birth assistant or their mother for support and resistance while pushing.

Parenting Tip If you're planning to breast-feed, it's a good idea to **take a front-buttoning nightgown or pullover pajama with you to the hospital or birth center or have one available to put on after home birth.** A pullover-style top is convenient because there are no buttons, it stays in place, and it's easy to see how your baby is doing.

Did You Know? Both goat's milk and cow's milk are poor sources of vitamin C, but **vitamin C is supplied generously by the breast milk of a well-nourished mother.**

DAY 177	DATE:
	89 days to go

By now, the baby's body is composed of **2 to 3 percent body fat.**

From time to time, you might experience some **pelvic pain** as your uterus grows and stretches the ligaments. Most often, the pain is felt in the groin area and inside your thighs, especially after you walk or exercise. Resting should bring you some relief.

Childbirth in Other Cultures The traditional Sirionó women of Bolivia gave birth in a hut crowded with other women, but no one typically offered any help. The laboring woman rested in a hammock slung low to the ground, and when the baby was born, he or she was actually allowed to slip out of the hammock and fall onto the ground, ostensibly to encourage baby to breathe!

Ready to Breast-Feed **A nursing stool is a footrest** that is angled to support your feet, legs, and ultimately your back while you sit to breast-feed or hold your baby. Some are adjustable while others are not. (If you are petite, you may already know what a difference a footrest can make in terms of comfort.)

One of the virtues of being very young is that you don't let the facts get in the way of your imagination.
SAM LEVENSON

DAY 178

DATE:

88 days to go

 Your **baby's eyelids begin to unfuse** and open partially.

Sometimes perspiration trapped in the folds of your skin can cause irritation. Such irritation is most noticeable in the pelvic area and under your breasts. Natural lotions and skin washes without fragrance and harsh chemicals can both cleanse and soothe.

Childbirth in Other Cultures Recorded in the papyrus of ancient Egypt (1900–1550 BCE) are instructions for calculating a pregnant woman's expected due date between 271 and 294 days from the onset of her LMP. The modern count is 280 days.

Ready to Breast-Feed **You might want to buy extra parts for your breast pump** so that one set can be soaking in soapy water while the other is being used.

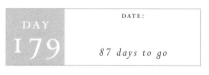

DAY 179

DATE:

87 days to go

In the next day or so, your **baby's eyes** will be completely formed as all of the cells have finished migrating to their correct locations. The **lashes** are beginning to appear.

You may have more **swelling** in your hands and feet now.

IMPORTANT: Avoid standing. Rest with your legs elevated. Both of these precautions will reduce swelling.

Parenting Tip Crying causes babies to swallow air, not the other way around. As long as he or she isn't ill, using a combination of **effective soothing strategies** can help. Try swaddling, rocking or swinging, non-nutritive sucking, and laying baby on his or her side or stomach. Every baby is different, so good luck!

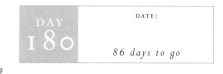

DAY 180

DATE:

86 days to go

The baby's **sucking and swallowing skills** are becoming more coordinated.

During pregnancy, a number of conditions can cause **fainting**: hot weather, sudden changes in posture, standing for long periods of time, fatigue, excitement, stress, stuffy rooms, and crowds.

Childbirth in Other Cultures In many cultures, older women are responsible for attending to women during childbirth. Some cultures designate certain women to be midwives; others assign the task to female relatives. Men may or may not be allowed in the room with the laboring women.

Parenting Tip **A safety seat for the car is one of the *most important* items you will ever purchase.** Here are some important questions to consider: What types of safety claims do the manufacturers make? Does the seat grow with your baby? Is it easy to keep clean? In most areas, law enforcement and fire departments will install it for you.

Chart your waist size and weight here and on page 182.

WAIST SIZE   WEIGHT

Hold a hand that needs you and discover abundant joy.

FLAVIA

DAY 181	DATE: *85 days to go*

By today or tomorrow, **eyelashes** are fully present on your baby's eyelids.

One of the most important things you'll need to do when you breast-feed is learn to relax. Relaxation allows your milk to flow. Select a quiet place to breast-feed. Be sure it is free from distractions (and without a clock to make you feel rushed). Your baby will stop nursing when he or she is full. Sometimes feeding sessions take a little longer, and sometimes they move a little more quickly. It will be unpredictable at first.

Did You Know? **At birth, a major valve must close inside the baby's heart** to keep the used blood and the fresh, oxygenated blood separated.

Parenting Tip You might want to prepare a low-fat snack and beverage for yourself to eat during the baby's nighttime feedings. **Baby may not be the only one who's hungry and you need to replenish your fluids!**

What do you want to be sure to remember?

_____

_____

_____

_____

_____

_____

_____

(See page 137 for more space to write.)

DAY 182	DATE: *84 days to go*

Today, as Week 26 comes to a close, your baby measures almost 10 inches (254 mm) in length and weighs 2⅛ lb (952 g). **In just two weeks, your baby has gained 6 oz (168 g)— nearly half a pound—and has grown ¾ inch (19.1 mm)!**

Your uterus continues to push on your bladder, reducing its capacity. During pregnancy, the tubes that lead from the kidneys to the bladder lack tone and are more readily stretched open, kinked, and compressed. **Thus, even with a smaller capacity, the bladder often can't be emptied fully, and urinary tract infection can result.**

For Your Comfort Since the muscles of your pelvic floor may not be able to prevent leakage when you laugh, cough, or strain to lift something, empty your bladder often.

Ready to Breast-Feed **You'll need to purchase baby bottles** in order to store expressed breast milk and to use with formula. Many of the baby bottles that you'll see advertised have their own specialized vented systems for keeping the baby from gulping air, for example. Ask your girlfriends about their experiences. Claims on commercial packaging can be misleading. But one thing is for sure—use glass or BPA-free plastic bottles.

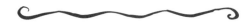

It is a wise father that knows his own child.

WILLIAM SHAKESPEARE

TIME TO REFLECT:

What's the most important thing you've learned about pregnancy so far?

_____

_____

_____

_____

_____

DAY 183

DATE:

83 days to go

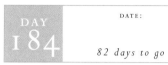 Your baby's eyes are sensitive to various levels of light and darkness but can't detect the outline of objects yet. Since light waves carry visual information to your baby's brain, **the baby's eyes are preparing to see after birth.**

Pregnancy is one of the three biological periods in a woman's life when her ability to cope with the emotional experiences of life can be more challenging. The other two times are at puberty and menopause. There is much individual variation from woman to woman influenced by biological factors like hormones, personality, social circumstances, psychological factors, and emotional reactivity.

Childbirth in Other Cultures In the Yucatán Peninsula, usually only the midwife, husband, and pregnant woman's mother are present at a birth. If the labor is long and difficult, other women will appear: mother-in-law, sisters, godmother, sisters-in-law, close friends, and neighbors.

DAY 184

DATE:

82 days to go

This is another highly significant day in your baby's development. The baby's brain can now direct rhythmic breathing and better control his or her body temperature.

This means that if your baby is born now, his or her brain can usually stimulate breathing and sustain that activity without medical intervention. It also means that the baby's body can help regulate its own temperature, taking steps to cool down when too warm or to warm up when too cold.

Childbirth in Other Cultures In most cultures, a new mother is encouraged to nurse her baby right away. **Colostrum, or premilk, contains more antibodies, proteins, and certain minerals than mature milk.** Breast milk itself is the perfect food since it **provides needed nutrients in** *exactly* **the right proportions.** The protein in breast milk is easily accessible to the newborn's system and acts as an antibacterial agent. That's why **breast-fed infants experience less vomiting, diarrhea, and ear infections than formula-fed babies.**

Ready to Breast-Feed **Nipple soreness** is especially common in the early weeks of breast-feeding, even if your baby is positioned correctly. Most importantly: **1.** Keep your nipples clean. **2.** Smooth 100 percent lanolin and expressed breast milk over your entire nipple after every feeding. The lanolin encourages moist healing and the breast milk has natural antibiotic properties.

It is a wise child that knows his own father.

HOMER

DAY
185
DATE:

81 days to go

Each day that passes brings your baby closer to birth and closer to completing the prenatal phase of his or her development. **The baby's ability to thrive outside your womb improves with each passing day.**

Your uterus goes from weighing 2 oz (56 g) to nearly 2¼ lbs (986 g) by the end of your pregnancy. This month, your weekly **weight gain should taper off** to ¾ lb (336 g) and then next month to ½ lb (224 g).

Childbirth in Other Cultures Among the peoples living in the Yucatán Peninsula, the woman's husband is traditionally expected to be present during her labor and childbirth. The culture says he should see how a woman suffers. This rule is quite stringent, and absent husbands are blamed for poor birth outcomes.

Feeding Your Baby **The composition of the milk changes to meet the changing energy and nutrient needs of your baby as he or she grows and develops.** For example, milk from a mother who gave birth prematurely meets the baby's developmental needs more completely than the milk from a mother who gave birth to a full-term infant. In short, the mother's body "knows" what to offer its newborn. How great is that?

Chart your waist size and weight here and on page 182.

WAIST SIZE   WEIGHT

DAY
186
DATE:

80 days to go

Over the next three days or so, **your baby's skin will become smoother** and less wrinkled as more fat is deposited underneath its surface.

Your blood pressure may begin to rise somewhat during this month. Slight increases are considered normal.

Contact your practitioner *immediately* **if you experience severe headaches, blurry vision, sudden weight gain, or severe swelling in the hands, feet, ankles, or face.** These symptoms can indicate high blood pressure, which can be dangerous for both you and your baby.

Ready to Breast-Feed The calcium-to-phosphorus ratio in **breast milk is ideal** for moving calcium into your baby's skeleton and promoting growth; the calcium in fortified soy milk isn't as bioavailable. In addition, the iron and zinc from breast milk are absorbed better than from formula derived from cow's milk.

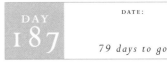

DAY
187
DATE:

79 days to go

Over the next three days, the **baby will become more sensitive to light, sound, taste, and smell.** The touch sensitivity of your baby's skin is already well established.

Your baby's body is preparing to see you, hear your voice, recognize you by your distinctive smell, and taste the liquid nutrition you will provide. **Imagine what you will say to your baby when the two of you meet and how you will stroke its skin and hold its tiny hand. Your baby's birth is not very far away.**

The world talks to the mind. Parents speak more intimately—they talk to the heart.
HAIM GINOTT

Did You Know? **Each square inch of the baby's skin** will ultimately contain 700 sweat glands, 100 oil-bearing glands, and 21,000 cells sensitive to heat!

Feeding Your Baby When breast-feeding, **second-time mothers with toddlers** have the challenge of keeping baby on the breast while supervising and tending to their toddler. If your firstborn is very busy and hard to keep occupied during the baby's feedings, you may find it easier to use a breast pump and bottle feed expressed milk or plan quicker, but more frequent, nursing.

Parenting Tip Use hot, soapy water and a bottle brush to **rinse out baby bottles, nipples, and rings immediately after use.** Again, use glass or BPA-free plastic bottles. BPA is a dangerous chemical that acts like the hormone estrogen in the environment. If the bottles are dishwasher safe, stack them upside down on the top rack to sterilize them. Bacteria from dirt or old milk can make your baby sick.

Childbirth in Other Cultures Aymara mothers of Brazil customarily take their new babies with them wherever they go. They also sleep with their babies for the first two years of life.

Feeding Your Baby Milk production burns between 500 and 650 calories per day—that's more than a pound per week because of breast-feeding alone. Thus, **weight loss is accelerated among women who breast-feed or combine breast-feeding with formula feeding for three months or longer.**

Ready to Breast-Feed Some Americans, breast-feeding moms included, feel uncomfortable with the idea of breast-feeding in public. In some areas, laws have been passed to protect moms who breast-feed from being arrested for indecent exposure! Whether you breast-feed in a women's lounge, beneath a blanket or wrap, or just let it all hang out, **we should congratulate our nursing mothers for giving their babies' brains and bodies the very best and encourage all moms to breast-feed!**

DAY 188	DATE:
	78 days to go

By today, **the surface of your baby's skin is smoother, brighter, and less red**, as body fat accumulates under its surface. The fat your baby is putting on is white fat, not brown fat that was used in temperature regulation earlier in the pregnancy. White fat is insulating and is an energy source. Fat babies aren't necessarily healthier babies, but some fat is needed for normal body functioning. The bladder is usually a round organ, but is flattened from external pressure during pregnancy. Thus, its retention capacity is greatly reduced.

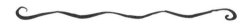

TIME TO REFLECT
What's the most important thing you've learned about yourself thus far?

Only love can be divided endlessly and still not diminish.
ANNE MORROW LINDBERGH

DAY
189

DATE:

77 days to go

The baby's eyes can now move in their sockets. **Your baby is practicing looking.** What does the baby "see"? Imagine for a moment what the inside of the womb must look like. Under bright lights or sunlight and without the protection of your clothing, the baby's world might look pinkish as the light shines through your blood vessels. At night, with clothing, or in a darkened room, it must be dark. The baby's system probably notices changes in light intensity. **But the color "pink" is a sensation that will take months to perceive.**

Childbirth in Other Cultures In many cultures, there are taboos against intercourse during the time of breast-feeding. Among the Arapesh of Papua New Guinea, for example, tradition forbids intercourse until the baby takes its first steps.

Consider This Besides breast-feeding, can you think of any other **activity that burns between 500 and 650 calories per day** while you're sitting down, eating, and relaxing? ☺

Parenting Tip **Help your baby ease off to sleep** at night by bathing it just before feeding. A bath will help to warm and relax baby and eventually encourage more nighttime than daytime sleeping.

What do you want to be sure to remember?

(See page 137 for more space to write.)

Having a family is like having a bowling alley installed in your brain.
MARTIN MULL

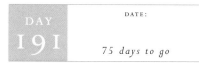

Week 28 Begins

LMP Week 30

DAY 190	DATE:
	76 days to go

Within the next three days, your baby's brain begins to take on a more wrinkled appearance because of its rapid growth. The wrinkling of the surface of the brain is normal and necessary. The wrinkles are called convolutions. **A convoluted brain contains more brain cells than a smooth, non-convoluted brain and is potentially much more powerful.**

Continue to identify any foods that don't seem to agree with you, and **avoid them**. These foods might include old favorites that have turned against you, new foods, or even foods you feel hungry for.

Childbirth in Other Cultures In Southeast Asia, a fire is lit in the traditional birthing hut to "roast" or "smoke" the new mother. The heat and smoke from the fire are thought to reduce soreness and to prevent the uterus from falling out of the mother.

IMPORTANT: Don't take anything for an upset stomach without first checking with your health-care provider.

Chart your waist size and weight here and on page 182.

WAIST SIZE   WEIGHT

DAY 191	DATE:
	75 days to go

Your baby will put on more than 1 lb (448 g) during this month. By the end of this week, baby's crown-to-rump length will be about 11 inches (28 cm)—**almost the size of a standard ruler.**

During this month, the **baby will actively absorb and store the nutrients you make available:** calcium for its developing skeleton, iron for its red blood cells, and protein for its growth.

From now on, your prenatal visits with your practitioner will take place every two weeks. It's important for your practitioner to keep tabs on how things are progressing as you come down to the final weeks. **Keep every appointment.**

Feeding Your Baby Pressure is produced inside the breast by the infant's sucking and the emptying of the breasts during a feeding. This causes a hormone to be released from the brain that stimulates the production of milk for the next feeding. **Only very rarely is a well-nourished, hydrated breast-feeding woman unable to produce enough milk for her baby.**

Parenting Tip At some point, every baby who will ever wear a diaper will have something that might be called diaper irritation or **diaper rash**. Have a product on hand that's made from natural ingredients and that works fast and effectively to relieve symptoms. Diaper rash is particularly common in baby's first 12 to 15 months. Consult with other moms to determine what works and what doesn't.

Never raise your hand to your children—it leaves your midsection unprotected.
ROBERT ORBEN

DAY 192

DATE:

74 days to go

By this time, **red blood cell production by the spleen ends and is entirely taken over by the bone marrow.** (Red blood cells were first produced by tissue groups called the blood islands, then by the liver, and after that by the spleen.) The spleen retains its potential for blood cell formation even into adulthood.

Air travel raises concerns about the impact of altitude change, dehydration, the difficulty of sitting for long periods of time in cramped quarters, the concern about swelling and blood clots, and the distance from medical care (both in the air and at your destination). Before you book airline tickets, discuss your plans with your health-care provider and the airline (some have specific policies).

Contact your practitioner if you feel you must travel by air during this time.

Did You Know? In preparation for milk production at birth, **each breast gains about 1 lb in fat and specialized tissue.** A healthy woman also adds 5 lb (2.3 kg) to the fat reserves in her body for lactation.

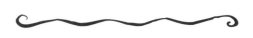

TIME TO REFLECT

What's the most important personality trait your child can possess?

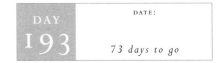

DAY 193

DATE:

73 days to go

Since the baby's eyelids are now unfused, they can both open and close. Much of the time, your baby's eyes are open and practicing "looking" movements.

You may experience **some pain and tenderness in the rib area right below your breasts** if the baby sits high in your uterus (pain is also due to frequent kicking).

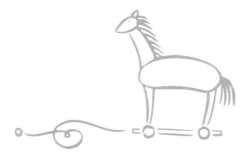

To be in your children's memories tomorrow, you have to be in their lives today.
ANONYMOUS

For Your Comfort You can **relieve some of the rib area discomfort** by lying down when you can and avoiding bending forward. The baby will begin to shift position and settle more into your pelvis as the pregnancy continues.

IMPORTANT: All babies under the age of one year should be placed flat on their backs to sleep. Babies placed face down can suffocate with pillows, plush animals, and fluffy bedding whether or not they can turn their heads. Some babies have brains that are not mature enough to reliably wake them up if they stop breathing. This tendency seems to be one factor associated with SIDS or Sudden Infant Death Syndrome, the leading cause of death in babies during their first year. **Remember, Back to Sleep** seems safest.

Ready to Breast-Feed **It looks like breast milk provides your baby with greater immune protection (fewer infections) and some protection against intestinal damage, breast cancer, cancer of the lymph nodes (lymphoma), childhood obesity, childhood-onset diabetes, and possibly even SIDS (Sudden Infant Death Syndrome).**

Parenting Tip **Try to establish a sleep routine** from the beginning, so the baby can anticipate going to sleep at a particular time. Sing the same song each time, rub the baby in a special spot only at bedtime, recite a particular rhyme or prayer, rock him or her, etc. This routine will be especially helpful when you're away from home and the baby needs to rest.

DAY 194	DATE:
	72 days to go

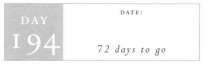 The process of myelinization begins to **speed nerve cell transmission.** *Myelin* is a fatty substance that coats the outside of nerve cells and makes nerve cell transmission faster, easier, and more efficient.

When you **sleep**, you may notice some discomfort due to indigestion or to the pressure of the baby and your uterus on your ribs and diaphragm.

For Your Comfort Try shifting positions to release the pressure due to indigestion, and avoid eating right before bedtime. Raising the head of the bed or having an extra pillow may help.

DAY 195	DATE:
	71 days to go

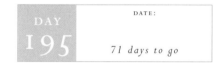 By now, most of the *lanugo* (the downy **hair that covered your baby's body**) has disappeared except for patches on the back and shoulders. However, the white (as yet unpigmented) **hair on your baby's head** is well developed.

You have probably noticed that the whitish **vaginal discharge has gotten heavier.** This is normal.

Contact your practitioner if the vaginal discharge is discolored or thick or is accompanied by symptoms of discomfort (pain, burning, itching), bleeding, or unusual odor.

Blessed are the young, for they shall inherit the national debt.
HERBERT HOOVER

Feeding Your Baby Feed the baby in as **upright** a position as possible. The bubble at the bottom of the baby's stomach will rise and be burped out easily, preventing the pain of trapped air in its stomach.

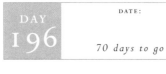

DAY
196

DATE:

70 days to go

Your baby's **toenails** may be visible.

When this day ends, you will have been **pregnant for seven complete months.**

Did You Know? While the baby's growth has been rapid and sustained for many weeks, **its growth rate will begin to slow as the date of birth approaches.**

Ready to Breast-Feed Moms who breast-feed need good support for their breasts to manage back pain. Check out the styles of nursing bras and ask the opinion of other nursing moms. (The ones you buy might look gigantic, but you'll find that they just barely fit when the time comes!)

What do you want to be sure to remember?

(See page 137 for more space to write.)

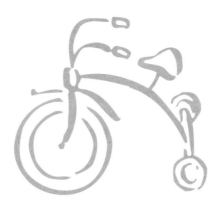

A babe is fed with milk and praise.

CHARLES LAMB

What do you want to remember about your **Seventh Month**?

(See pages 187 to 192 for entering labor and delivery details.)

Lunar Month 8

THINGS TO DO THIS MONTH:

* Take steps to control heartburn.

* Check out breast-feeding resources on the Web.

* Begin to gather bottle-feeding supplies (even if you will begin by breast-feeding).

* Consider using a baby carrier; look at different styles.

* Install night-lights or dimmer switches in your home for safer nighttime feedings.

* Use breast pads if your breasts are starting to leak.

* Don't scratch itchy skin, soothe it.

* Get help with preparing for your baby's first weeks.

* Put together two prepared bags—one for the baby and one for you (if you'll be giving birth away from home).

* Get back on track if you've fallen away from your healthy habits.

Week 29 Begins

DAY	DATE:
197	*69 days to go*

Your baby's **crown-to-rump measurement** is now about 11 inches (280 mm). His or her weight is at least 2¾ lb (1,300 g), the weight of a quart and a half of water!

Your uterus has expanded to a point halfway between your navel and the end of your breastbone. If you are experiencing digestive tract discomforts or are having trouble inhaling and fully inflating your lungs, that's probably why!

Your practitioner may order more blood tests for you sometime during this month to make sure your pregnancy is progressing well.

For Your Comfort Here are some **more ideas to help with heartburn**: **1.** Don't overeat—instead, eat several small meals a day. **2.** Don't go to bed or lie down until two to three hours after eating. **3.** Drink fluids mostly between meals, not with your meal.

Parenting Tip **If you need extra bedrest after the birth** (as women with difficult births and C-sections often do), make the bed a playpen and baby-care station by keeping toys, books, diapers, clothing, food, and items needed for breast-feeding within reach. Better yet, get some temporary help with caring for the baby so you can rest and recuperate. Right after the baby is born, use disposable plates and cups, and order healthy takeout to minimize preparation and cleanup.

DAY	DATE:
198	*68 days to go*

Your baby's growth in height and weight will slow between now and birth. Even so, your **baby will gain about 2 lb (896 g) this month!**

If you haven't already, you might want to **investigate online breast-feeding resources** that make it easier for first-time moms and mothers of children who haven't breast-fed before. For example, the specialists who staff the Office of Women's Health (www.womenshealth.gov/breast-feeding) offer guidance and training. La Leche League International (www.lalecheleague.org) has more than 50 years of service teaching ALL women what they call "The Womanly Art of Breast-Feeding."

Did You Know? **Your baby's brain is now so sophisticated that if it were born today, it could see, hear, remember, and learn.** Scientists believe that the presence of these brain activities marks the beginning of true consciousness, since the baby's brain exhibits all of the brain waves (although not in the same sequence) that an adult brain exhibits.

Parenting Tip If you use a soft-fabric front carrier like a sling, let the infant sleep upright occasionally if you are comfortable doing so.

Unlike grown-ups, children have little need to deceive themselves.

J. W. GOETHE

DAY 199	DATE:
	67 days to go

If your baby is born now, **it may have a callous on its thumb from sucking it** in the womb.

Cavities in your teeth during pregnancy are more often caused by a slight decrease in the pH of the saliva or by inadequate brushing, flossing, or dental care than by any pregnancy-induced changes in the teeth themselves.

IMPORTANT: While your baby isn't growing much bigger in ways that can be easily measured, its internal systems and tissues continue to become more sophisticated. For those reasons, the **calcium, protein, iron, B-complex vitamins, zinc, vitamin A, and folic acid in your diet continue to be very important.**

Feeding Your Baby Freeze any expressed breast milk that won't be used immediately. Thaw frozen breast milk gently in warm water, but never by microwaving (it destroys the antibodies). For safe handling, do not refreeze thawed breast milk.

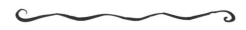

TIME TO REFLECT
If there's one thing you could change about your life right now, what would it be?

DAY 200	DATE:
	66 days to go

For about the last month, your baby has assumed the fetal position in your uterus. **The legs have been drawn in to the chest because there isn't room for them to straighten out.**

You will continue to notice strong, methodical activity from the baby. **It might seem as though the baby is more active at night** than at other times. This may be the case, but it may also be that you simply notice the movements more because you are less distracted by other things.

Ready to Breast-Feed Breast milk is a natural food abundant with immune protection and healthy phytonutrients and antioxidants. **I'll say it again: There is no better nutrition on the planet than the milk from a healthy mom, especially if the baby was born early.** That's because breast milk is a dynamic fluid whose composition changes over time according to infant needs. Your body "remembers" when your baby was born and produces just the right blend of nutrients for each developmental age.

Consider This The Surgeon General of the United States recommends that **babies drink only breast milk** for the first six months because that's what they *need*. Happily, 79 percent of newborns begin breast-feeding, but only half are still receiving breast milk by the time they are six months old. There is a variety of reasons why babies are weaned from the breast, but try to stay with it just as long as you are able. Breast milk enhances intelligence!

They are idols of hearts and households; / They are angels of God in disguise; / The sunlight still sleeps in their tresses; / His glory still gleams in their eyes.

CHARLES DICKENS

DAY 201	DATE:
	65 days to go

There are four layers of tissue in the placenta separating your blood supply from your baby's. **Unless some breakdown of the placenta occurs, the baby's blood never mixes with yours.**

You may notice that you're a little **clumsy** these days. This is due to the increased size of your uterus, the loosening of your joints to prepare for childbirth, and the shifts in the baby's position.

If you fall, contact your practitioner *immediately* so she can ask you about any other symptoms you might be experiencing.

Did You Know? Take care not to lose your balance but, if you do, remember that the **baby is protected by one of the most efficient shock-minimizing systems on earth**—the amniotic fluid contained in your tough, muscular uterus!

Consider This Holding on to the handle of a sturdy baby carrier or the rails of a treadmill while you exercise by walking may be prudent. So would be placing a hand on the back of a chair to steady yourself while stretching or practicing balancing exercises. If the weather is nice, swimming can feel wonderful, but **move slowly** in and out of the pool and watch for slippery surfaces.

Chart your waist size and weight here and on page 182.

WAIST SIZE   WEIGHT

DAY 202	DATE:
	64 days to go

The baby's brain is still developing rapidly, increasing the number of interconnections between individual nerve cells and identifying groups of cells that will perform complicated functions throughout your baby's lifetime.

As your uterus continues to stretch these final weeks, **your abdomen may ache more.**

For Your Comfort **Try to rest and get off your feet.** A heating pad and supportive pillows may help relieve achiness.

Ready to Breast-Feed **Synthetic versions of two essential fats found naturally in breast milk**—DHA (docosahexaenoic acid) and ARA (arachidonic acid)—have been added to almost all brands of infant formula to maintain a balance of fatty acids. Formula with these supplements claims to support the development of brain cells and vision. As of this writing, no study has shown that the synthetic fatty acids are as effective in supporting development as their natural counterparts in human milk; in fact, they may be associated with side effects. If you stop breast-feeding and can't wean your baby onto a cup, ask your practitioner for advice.

For Your Information **Breast milk** contains hundreds of components that as yet cannot be copied and added to baby formula. These natural substances seem to offer unrivaled immune protection against illness.

Parenting Tip **Put the baby down when it is drowsy** but still awake, so it will learn to drift off to sleep without help from you.

Sweet babe, in thy face / Soft desires I can trace, / Secret joys and secret smiles, / Little pretty infant wiles.
WILLIAM BLAKE

DATE:

DAY

2 0 3

63 days to go

Sometime between now and Week 40, the baby's testes will have completely descended, if it's a boy. To review, the testes are formed in the body cavity from the same tissue that forms the female baby's ovaries. While the female's ovaries descend to a position just below the brim of the pelvis, **the body cavity is too warm for the male's testes and their sperm-producing mechanisms. Eventually, the testes migrate into the scrotum.** In the scrotum, the tissue of the temperature-sensitive testes can be perfectly maintained by bringing them closer to the body to warm them or relaxing the muscles to distance them from the body and cool them.

Calcium needs are greatest during the last 12 weeks of your pregnancy, when rapid hardening of the baby's skeleton is taking place and calcium is required for bone development. The calcium in milk or milk products is very readily absorbed and utilized, while the calcium in pill form is not.

Did You Know? A total of **222 bones** is needed to adequately support the soft parts of the baby's body, especially during sitting and standing.

Childbirth in Other Cultures Historically, new mothers in Mexico are given steam baths after giving birth to help relieve pain and soreness.

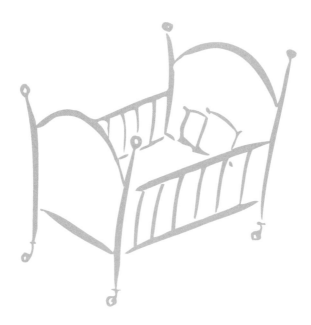

Sweet childish days, that were as long / As twenty days are now.
WILLIAM WORDSWORTH

DAY	DATE:
204	*62 days to go*

At this point, your baby can register information from **four of its five senses.**

This month, you may notice **some increased shortness of breath.** As the baby gets bigger and crowds more and more into your lungs, it's going to take more effort for you to breathe deeply. **Shortness of breath does not mean oxygen deprivation for you or the baby.**

Did You Know? At birth, your **baby's sense of touch** will be the most sensitive and well developed of all its senses.

Feeding Your Baby **The volume of breast milk produced depends more on how much milk the baby consumes** than on how much fluid the mother drinks. Nevertheless, fluid intake is important to protect against dehydration.

Parenting Tip Even though you can't use a baby carrier for as long as you can use a stroller, there are **some really good reasons to "wear your baby,"** not the least of which is having a comfortable support for breast-feeding.

What do you want to be sure to remember?

(See page 154 for more space to write.)

DAY	DATE:
205	*61 days to go*

While your baby's senses may be prepared to process information, certain senses have limited opportunities to operate. Since the baby doesn't breathe air inside your uterus, **the sense of smell is on hold until after birth.**

As the baby's arrival approaches, your body is going to spend more and more time practicing for the birth. Specifically, **the muscles of your uterus will practice contracting and relaxing.**

Did You Know? Practice contractions are called Braxton-Hicks contractions. They are **generally painless** but may be experienced more frequently from now on.

Feeding Your Baby **Women who have concerns about breast-feeding in front of others** should consider expressing (or pumping) their breast milk and transferring it to a bottle for feeding. **In that way, the baby gets all the benefits of its mother's milk and the mother can avoid situations that may be potentially uncomfortable.**

Ready to Breast-Feed The benefits of therapeutic medications taken by the mother should always be weighed against the risks before breast-feeding. Drugs present in your system will almost always be present in your breastmilk to some degree, most at low levels. **Your practitioner can evaluate each medication** to determine which pose no real risk to most infants, recommend a safer alternative, or advise breast-feeding when the meds are at lower levels in your milk.

The sweetest flowers in all the world—/ A baby's hands.

ALGERNON CHARLES SWINBURNE

DAY 2 06	DATE:
	60 days to go

The colored portion, or iris, of your baby's eye is beginning to respond to the intensity of the light by opening under dim light conditions and closing under bright light conditions. This activity is automatic and is called the pupillary reflex.

Weak abdominal muscles can cause a woman to hold her shoulders too far back in order to support her uterus. The resulting muscle strain leads to fatigue and back pain. Exercise regularly.

If you have any concerns about the contractions you may be experiencing—or you think you might actually be going into labor—give your practitioner a call. Don't go to the hospital or the emergency room. Ask your practitioner's advice first.

Parenting Tip To make nighttime baby checks easier, put a dimmer on the light switch, keep a flashlight handy, or turn on a few energy-efficient night-lights.

DAY 2 07	DATE:
	59 days to go

Within the next three days, your **baby's toenails** will be fully formed.

This month **you will notice many of the same symptoms you've experienced before**, including backaches. The small of your back will have an increasingly difficult time balancing the load, as you and the baby get larger.

If your backache is severe and persistent, contact your practitioner.

Parenting Tip Remember to burp your baby with each feeding. Air that gets trapped in the stomach during feeding can cause discomfort and regurgitation. Patting can be firm, just not jarring. Also, if you've given burping a good try and you don't get anything, that's okay. If the baby seems comfortable, no worries.

Chart your waist size and weight here and on page 182.

WAIST SIZE   WEIGHT

DAY 2 08	DATE:
	58 days to go

The hair on your baby's head is growing longer. Depending on the genetic tendencies in your family and that of the baby's father, your baby will either be born with a full head of hair or a very sparse hair pattern on its scalp. Both are completely normal.

You may continue to have **leg cramps**, especially when you are trying to sleep.

If leg soreness and pain persist, contact your practitioner so the possibility of a blood clot in your leg can be ruled out.

Did You Know? The circulating hormones that are preparing your breasts for milk production **also cause the mammary glands in your baby's breasts to swell.** You will probably notice this temporary effect at birth whether your baby is male or female. Breast tissue swelling is normal; the tissue will shrink back within several days after birth.

The thing about having a baby is that thereafter you have it.

JEAN KERR

Ready to Breast-Feed The **amount of breast milk produced** by a breast-feeding mother varies from woman to woman. The average at first is about 1 cup (235 mL), doubling to 2 cups (470 mL) by day seven, and 4 cups (940 mL) by two weeks. Remember to drink lots of water while the baby feeds.

DAY 209	DATE:
	57 days to go

 By today, your baby's toenails will be fully formed. If your baby is a boy, his testes are still making their descent into the scrotum.

You may notice some colostrum leaking from your breasts—it's a yellowish fluid that precedes actual milk production. Colostrum is your baby's first natural food. It's a superfood that is rich in antibodies and protects your baby from middle-ear infection, respiratory illness, diarrhea, breast cancer, intestinal disorders like Crohn's disease, staph infection, the flu, and more.

Childbirth in Other Cultures By tradition, some new mothers in the Philippines are given a special meal after childbirth of boiled chicken, corn porridge, and a small amount of cooked placenta.

Parenting Tip Use a handheld **shower hose** or even the kitchen **sink sprayer** when bathing a baby in a baby tub. The baby will enjoy the feel of the running water, and you can wash and rinse the whole body easily—even the hair. Never let the baby hold the sprayer by himself. Not only will baby make a big mess, but he or she may also direct the spray into his or her face and risk inhaling the water.

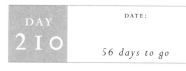

DAY 210	DATE:
	56 days to go

Because of the rapid brain growth of the last few weeks, **the circumference of your baby's head has increased** by about ⅜ inch (9.5 mm). The developing brain pushes outward on the skull, but it also folds in upon itself to create more of the convolutions mentioned earlier.

Mild swelling of your hands, feet, ankles, and face is still considered to be common, as excess fluid continues to collect in your tissues.

For Your Comfort Drinking plenty of fluids, elevating your legs when you sit, lying on your left side, trying to maintain a comfortable body temperature, and wearing support stockings can **all help you feel more comfortable.**

Parenting Tip Keep disposable gloves on your hands for a better grip when holding and washing your baby. **Wet babies are as slippery as little fish!**

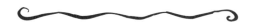

TIME TO REFLECT
What tasks do you need to accomplish before your baby is born?

_____

_____

_____

_____

The mother-child relationship is paradoxical and, in a sense, tragic.
It requires the most intense love on the mother's side, yet this very love must help the child
grow away from the mother and to become fully independent.
ERICH FROMM

LMP Week 33

DAY 2 I I	DATE:
	55 days to go

DAY 2 I 2	DATE:
	54 days to go

As you begin Week 31, **your baby is con- tinuing to grow at an amazing rate.** Right now, he measures around a foot (305 mm) long and weighs about 3 to 3¾ lb (1,700 g—the weight equivalent of 7 cups of water). By the time this week ends, your baby will have added almost ⅜ inch (9.5 mm) to its length!

As I've said all along, **the placenta is a very complex and complete organ.** Every enzyme known to exist in biology (except ACTH) has been found in the placenta. That means the placenta can play a role in any hormonal process that affects growth, sexual development, and the breakdown of nutrients into energy to fuel prepara- tion for birth.

Parenting Tip If you're bottle-feeding, measure out the amount of formula powder needed for a single serving. Put aside six or eight individual portions into segmented plastic containers or baggies to use when it's dark or you're tired **so that you won't risk overnourishing or undernourishing the baby.**

Depending on its size and position in your uterus, the baby may be carried high (pressed up against your lungs) or low (pressing against your pelvis); your baby may lie in a position that makes you look wide or compact; and you may look bigger or smaller than women who are just as far along as you with their pregnancies.

You may be bothered more by consti- pation now than before. As your uterus becomes larger, it pushes more on your bowel, inter- fering with its normal activity and making it more sluggish than usual.

Ready to Breast-Feed While "breast is best" for infant nutrition, especially if your baby is born prematurely or is ill, **there are cases where human milk is not recommended.** Practitioners take the mother's medical condition, treatments, and habits— especially drug, alcohol, tobacco, and marijuana use—into account when weighing the balance of risk to benefit of using her breast milk.

Parenting Tip If your older child asks to try breast- feeding, whether he or she gets a turn or not depends entirely on you. Allowing your child to (re)experience nursing will satisfy his curiosity in a way that reminding him about his babyhood won't. And if you like, you can say once is enough. Remember, your breasts will replace any milk that is produced, so you don't have to worry about "running out." **Handle this issue in the way that feels most comfortable to you without shaming your child.**

Your children will become what you are, so be what you want them to be.

DAVID BLY

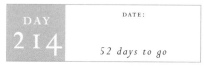

DAY 213

DATE:

53 days to go

By about this point, the volume of amniotic fluid has reached its maximum. **As your baby grows, there will be less fluid and more baby and thus, you will feel considerably more movement from within.** The amniotic fluid is clear, watery, and straw-colored. By the time you reach your delivery date, the amniotic sac contains a full liter of fluid.

Your breasts will feel increasingly nodular or lumpy as they prepare for milk production. **Breast changes will be most noticeable if this is your first pregnancy.**

Did You Know? Eighty percent of the cells in breast milk are specialized for killing fungi, viruses, and bacteria. **Amazing natural protection for your little one!**

For Your Comfort Stretching skin on your abdomen and breasts means itchy skin. **Try not to scratch,** even though you might be tempted to do so. **Check with your practitioner for anti-itch suggestions; swimming can be soothing.**

What do you want to be sure to remember?

(See page 154 for more space to write.)

DAY 214

DATE:

52 days to go

Sometimes babies at this stage **practice sucking** by sucking their thumbs or fingers (their quarters are too cramped for them to reach their toes!).

Although you may be quite tired, **you still may have difficulty sleeping** because of backache, baby movement, feeling too hot, headaches, leg cramps, or trouble finding a comfortable position.

IMPORTANT: Remember that when you lie down, try always to **roll to your left side** (it improves your circulation and the baby's and aids in your digestion and breathing). If you haven't already tried a full body pillow, you might consider something similar now.

Parenting Tip **If you work outside the home,** think about how to balance your life with the addition of the new baby. Planning your working life around a second child is significantly different from planning for the first because it is infinitely more complicated. There is at least twice as much to do, if not more. Two children with two different personalities and (sometimes) two destinations—school for the older child and day care for the younger—make working a challenge, particularly for single moms and women with little job flexibility.

The world will never get any better until children are an improvement on their parents.

BOB EDWARDS

DAY	DATE:
215	*51 days to go*

Your baby is about 1 inch (25.4 mm) **longer than it was just four days ago!**

You may notice more leg fatigue and more varicose veins in your legs and abdomen. As your weight and blood volume increase, more and more pressure is placed on the veins of your legs and the legs themselves, resulting in a dull, aching pain.

For Your Comfort Try putting on **support stockings** as soon as you get up in the morning to ease the achiness. Also, **stay off your feet** as much as possible.

Parenting Tip How can you merge motherhood with working outside the home? For some women, working part-time or quitting work is not an option. **Don't make any irrevocable decisions about work based on projection—wait until you've had the baby and you can better see what your new life is like.** Working is something that some women simply must do to be good mothers who feel happy and productive. Every woman has her own style, and, hopefully, you will be able to structure your life the way you need it to be, whether it involves working outside the home or not.

Chart your waist size and weight here and on page 182.

WAIST SIZE   WEIGHT

DAY	DATE:
216	*50 days to go*

As fat accumulates under the baby's skin, his or her **skin color changes from dark red and transparent to pinkish and translucent** (even in babies who will eventually be dark-skinned). Your baby is making his or her greatest demands for protein and fat now during the last half of pregnancy. In the last six to eight weeks before birth, he or she will double in weight.

Some women are concerned about the **dreams** they have during pregnancy, but dreaming a lot is normal. When we go through transitional times in our lives—and pregnancy definitely qualifies as one—we have more worries and concerns than during the times we feel more stable. **Change, even a good change like having a baby, requires adjustment, and adjustment causes stress.** Worries you have during your waking hours (Will the baby be okay? Will I be a good parent? Can I handle the responsibility?) might also be examined when you dream, because they're still on your mind.

For Your Comfort **Rather than letting worry overtake you, try to confront your concerns.** If you're worrying about whether the baby will be healthy, take all the steps within your power to make sure you're doing the best you possibly can. If you still need to prepare for the baby's birth or first few weeks, write a to-do list and accomplish the easiest items first just to get you started. **Prioritize, delegate, organize, consult.** In addition, consider meditation, prayer, massage, exercise, or yoga as stress-control strategies.

List of parental requirements: Affection without sentiment, authority without cruelty, discipline without aggression, humor without ridicule, sacrifice without obligation, companionship without possessiveness.
WILLIAM E. BLATZ

DAY **217**	DATE: *49 days to go*

At the close of this week of pregnancy, the circumference, or distance around your baby's head has increased by about ⅜ inch (9.5 mm), due to **consistently rapid brain growth**.

Depending on the season of the year, it may be easier or more difficult for you to maintain a well-balanced diet. If it's winter, you might find you're hungrier, but the variety of foods isn't great. If it's summer, you may be less hungry because of the heat, but have more fresh fruits and vegetables available. ☺

For Your Health Whatever the time of year, **enjoy organically grown seasonal foods from local growers.** Sometimes finding new ways to prepare familiar fruits or vegetables makes them more interesting again.

Childbirth in Other Cultures After a child's birth, the traditional Tolong of the Philippines place the placenta in a clay pot, smoke it, and then bury the pot.

What do you want to be sure to remember?

(See page 154 for more space to write.)

TIME TO REFLECT

What's one thing that you have done for your baby every day without fail?

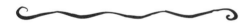

We are transfused into our children, and feel more keenly for them than for ourselves.

MARIE DE SÉVIGNÉ

Week 32 Begins

DAY 218	DATE:
	48 days to go

Your baby is still growing rapidly, and **underlying fat deposits are smoothing the appearance of the skin.** During this week, baby will grow ½ inch (13 mm) longer—about the diameter of a U.S. dime!

From this time on, your baby has some of the maturity needed to adapt to living outside the womb if born. This is reassuring news, especially since some babies apparently can't wait to leave their cramped quarters! Technically, though, **a month and a half of developmental progress awaits.**

Childbirth in Other Cultures In the Yucatán, massage (*sobada*) is part of each visit by the midwife. If any midwife determines that the baby is in a breech or transverse position, she may do an **inversion**, locating the baby's head and hip and applying strong, even pressure to rotate the baby's body into the more favorable head-down position. This is sometimes painful, but it is preferred over a Cesarean section.

Parenting Tip **You shouldn't expect a comfortable routine to develop quickly after the birth.** Adjusting to the needs and patterns of a new baby takes time, even if you've had other children. The baby's habits probably won't fit into the established routine, and expecting disruptions in the old order can make them easier to endure. Decide well before the birth who is responsible for certain chores so other family members can adapt with less confusion.

DAY 219	DATE:
	47 days to go

Your baby's eyes will open during the alert times of its daily cycle, and close when it sleeps. **The eyes are usually blue at this time, regardless of the final color they will become,** because the pigmentation that colors the eye is not fully developed. Final formation of eye pigmentation generally requires a few weeks' exposure to light.

Even though your baby's eyes can now process visual information, it's difficult to imagine what the baby's world must look like to it, especially since their focusing ability is poor. **Even after birth, babies are several weeks old before they can see their first color—red!**

Think About It The decision about **medication during labor** is an individual one. Being able to "tough it out" doesn't necessarily make you more dedicated or a better mother. If, after the onset of labor, you feel you want some type of pain relief, discuss your options with your practitioner. Pain medications administered during labor *do not* cause birth defects.

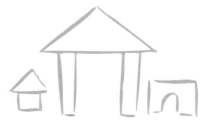

Pretty much all the honest truth telling there is in the world is done by children.

OLIVER WENDELL HOLMES

Parenting Tip **Keep a well-stocked diaper bag** near the front door that you can easily grab when you leave the house. Load it with diapers, an extra set of clothes, wipes, a light blanket, and waterproof bags. If you are breast-feeding, have a supply of natural nipple butter, compresses to help soothe sore breasts, and breast pads. If you are bottle-feeding, keep several clean bottle sets with dry formula in them and a bottle of clean water. Also pack a snack and water for yourself and your older child. Don't forget to restock the bag after your outing. Whew!

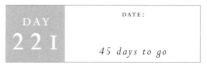

DAY 220	DATE:
	46 days to go

In addition to the immune protection provided by you, **your baby is also beginning to develop its own immune reaction to mild infections.**

Throughout your pregnancy, you have been supplying your baby with antibody protection to help make it immune to respiratory and gastrointestinal infections as well as to common viral infections (like measles), if such antibodies are present in your system. The antibodies are passed from your bloodstream through the placenta to the baby's bloodstream.

Talk with your practitioner about the best approach to successful breast-feeding.

Did You Know? **If you breast-feed your baby, antibodies will continue to be passed from you to your baby** and will continue to protect your child from disease. Although immunity cannot be acquired to whooping cough (pertussis) or chicken pox, **formula-fed babies receive *no* immune protection from the milk they drink.**

DAY 221	DATE:
	45 days to go

In the next three days, **the baby's fingernails will reach the ends of the fingertips.**

Most physicians don't recommend travel during the last two months of your pregnancy. Long trips by car are too exhausting; other modes of transportation place too much distance between you and your practitioner.

For Your Comfort If you need a **change of scenery,** take short trips until after the baby is born or get a big screen HDTV!

Did You Know? At birth, the **baby's umbilical cord** is closed naturally by a special jellylike substance that surrounds the vessels of the cord throughout pregnancy. The jelly swells up with exposure to the air and compresses the embedded vessels like a tourniquet. Some naturally occurring hormones in the jelly also help to prevent bleeding. **That's why when the cord is cut, it is practically bloodless.**

Easing the Transition from One Child to Two No matter how eagerly awaited the arrival of the second baby is, **the first child's life will always have to undergo a major change.** They now have to share every aspect of their existence with someone who seems to be getting more than his or her fair share of the parents' attention and affection. Some suggestions for easing the transition from one child to two or more will be offered over the next few weeks.

Children are poor men's riches.
ENGLISH PROVERB

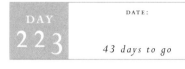

DAY	DATE:
222	*44 days to go*

Since **the amniotic fluid volume has reached its maximum**, you can now think of your baby as resting on the walls of your uterus rather than actually floating in a fluid-filled space. He or she is still bathed in amniotic fluid, of course, and that fluid is replaced continuously by your efficient system.

Within the next week or so, **your total blood volume will increase** in anticipation of the birth. The increased blood volume adds 2 to 4 lb (907 to 1,814 g) of weight. Whether you give birth vaginally or by Cesarean section, vitamin C, iron, zinc, and energy (one calorie is needed to produce one gram of collagen) are principally needed to help you heal.

Did You Know? The surface of the umbilical cord contains no pain receptors, so **cutting the cord at birth is not painful for the baby or you in any way.**

Parenting Tip If you breast-feed, you may find that your **breasts become engorged** sometimes and are quite uncomfortable. Try relieving the fullness in your breasts by expressing milk while taking a warm shower or bath if the baby isn't ready to nurse or if you're too sore to try. Milk flows better when you are warm. Breast pumps can also provide relief.

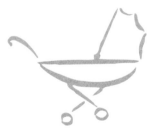

DAY	DATE:
223	*43 days to go*

By today, your baby's fingernails have reached the ends of her fingertips. You may find you have to cut his or her nails after birth. Even though the nails are small, they can still scratch (babies scratch themselves because of their poor muscle control). **The newborn's face may even have some scratch marks on it from his or her own long fingernails.**

At this point in the pregnancy, some women's **blood pressure may be rather unstable.** A slight drop in blood pressure can cause fainting, dizziness, and headaches.

IMPORTANT: 1. Change position slowly and deliberately (especially when getting up from lying flat). 2. Make sure your blood sugar doesn't drop too low (eat regularly). 3. Sit in well-ventilated areas. 4. Try to maintain a comfortable body temperature. 5. Drink plenty of water.

Childbirth in Other Cultures In many cultures, both ancient and current, the placenta is wrapped up and buried after the birth.

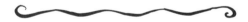

TIME TO REFLECT
What's one thing that your baby does for you every day?

_____

_____

_____

_____

_____

The rich don't have children; they have heirs.
PETER C. NEWMAN

Easing the Transition from One Child to Two Try not to imply that the baby needs you more than your firstborn does. **Everyone has different needs—** both immediate and long-term—and everyone has to learn to take turns. It's important to keep the turn-taking as fair as possible, and it's often necessary to give the older child even more lap time and affection than usual.

What do you want to be sure to remember?

_____

_____

_____

_____

_____

_____

(See page 154 for more space to write.)

DAY **224**	DATE:
	42 days to go

If your baby is born now, it will not only **be able to make an efficient transition from the womb to the outside,** but it will also be able to resist disease. Such a relief!

This day marks the end of eight months (32 weeks) of pregnancy. **You're heading for the home stretch!**

Did You Know? **Your baby's growth rate is still astonishing and requires every bit of your support.** Over the past week, his or her head circumference has increased by about another ⅜ inch (9.5 mm) due to its rapid brain development. **The critical period for the development of the baby's brain occurs in these last months of pregnancy.**

Parenting Tip Try to anticipate possible scenarios and prepare as much as you can for them. At this point, you should **consider the possibility that baby's birth may be premature**, and prioritize. If your baby were to come soon—say, within the next day or so—what do you still need to do to get ready? Is there unpacking, shopping, or organizing to do? Have you fallen out of a good habit—like drinking enough fluids each day—that you need to get back to? **Force yourself to establish priorities and systematically move through your to-do list.** There's no time like the present.

Easing the Transition from One Child to Two **Teach your oldest some child-care skills**, like how to hold or feed the baby, if he or she seems interested. Tell your oldest this is practice in case your older "baby" is a mommy or a daddy some day.

Chart your waist size and weight here and on page 182.

WAIST SIZE   WEIGHT

_____

Each time you look at your child you see something mysterious and contradictory—bits and pieces of other people—grandparents, your mate, yourself, all captured in a certain stance, a shape of a head, a look in the eyes, combined with something very precious—a new human soul rich in individuality and possibility.

JOAN SUTTON

What do you want to remember about your **Eighth Month?**

(See pages 187 to 192 for entering labor and delivery details.)

Lunar Month

Average pregnancy
lasts 9½ lunar months.
Lunar Month 10 actually
begins with Week 37.

THINGS TO DO THIS MONTH:

* If you are feeling forgetful, write down things you want to remember (instructions you get during check-ups, lists of things to do, and so on).

* Find answers to all your questions by consulting your health-care provider, lactation consultant, moms' group, etc.

* Begin to make your house baby-safe.

* Ask your practitioner about the absorption of herbal and cosmetic products for skin care.

* Try to relax and rest as much as possible.

* **Have a backup plan for everything.**

* Get ready to take and store pictures of your baby.

* Add the number of the American Association of Poison Control Centers (1-800-222-1222) to your list of phone contacts.

Good luck! You can do this!

Week 33 Begins

DAY 225	DATE: 41 days to go

Right now, your baby weighs at least 4½ lb (2,100 g) and measures almost 12 inches (300 mm) crown to rump. Baby's rapid growth **changes body proportions.** For example, the liver, which at Week 9 was 10 percent of baby's body weight, is now 5 percent of that total weight.

The lunar months of pregnancy are a little deceiving. Because each lunar month has four weeks of 7 days each (28 days total), **the baby actually requires 266 days, or nine and a half months, to complete development.**

Childbirth in Other Cultures By tradition, pregnant Arabic women would practice the dance that Westerners call "belly dancing" as a way of strengthening their abdominal muscles in preparation for childbirth. During labor, the mother was encircled by her fellow tribeswomen who danced by her bedside in an effort to "hypnotize" her into imitating the movements with her own body. The dance movements helped reduce the pain of labor and helped the mother work with her contractions to push the baby out.

Parenting Tip **Begin childproofing the house now** by moving all cleaning supplies from the spaces under sinks and cabinets and locking them in high, out-of-reach storage sites. Your baby will be crawling before you know it!

DAY 226	DATE: 40 days to go

If the baby is a boy, his testes will have finished descending sometime between now and his expected date of delivery. **The sperm-producing (seminiferous) tubules in your son's testes remain solid until puberty, at which time they begin to hollow out to produce sperm.**

Sometime within the next three days, your total blood volume will have increased from 17 to 21½ cups (4 to 5½ L) in preparation for birth. Twenty-one cups comes close to filling the space taken up by 10 lb of flour. **Blood loss during childbirth is inevitable since, among other things, the placenta has to separate from the uterine wall.** With a surplus of blood, some can be lost without undue risk. Continue to drink plenty of fluids, and get sufficient iron, calcium, copper, and vitamin K.

Childbirth in Other Cultures In cultures where women play an important role in the economic structure of the society, for example, in Tierra del Fuego, women must be separated from their babies soon after childbirth so they can return to their work and responsibilities.

Parenting Tip In the summer, cover your child's car seat with a sheet, towel, or blanket when not in use. **The seat can become very hot** and burn the baby's tender skin. Use a window shade or apply solar film to the windows in the back seat. **Park where it's shady.**

If, in instructing a child, you are vexed with it for want of adroitness, try, if you have never tried before, to write with your left hand, and then remember that a child is all left hands.

J. F. BOYSE

DAY 227	DATE:
	39 days to go

The baby might "drop" (settle down into your pelvis) before labor begins, but not all babies drop prior to the onset of labor.

If the baby drops (this is also called **settling or lightening**), you will begin to notice a decrease in lap space when seated, a sudden ease of breathing, more stomach capacity (since the load has shifted down), more pelvic pressure, and more frequent urination, maybe even difficulty holding your urine.

At each prenatal visit, your practitioner will check to see where the baby is positioned in your pelvis and will monitor your cervix for signs of dilation (widening) and effacement (thinning).

IMPORTANT: Be aware of these pelvic sensations, but don't worry if they aren't happening according to a set schedule. While dropping or settling is expected two to four weeks before delivery, it's hard to predict the events of birth. **Every baby has his or her own timetable.**

Easing the Transition from One Child to Two No matter how interested or capable your oldest seems, a child younger than 10 or 12 can't be expected to babysit. **A babysitter assumes full responsibility for the baby when you're not there**, and that's a job an adult needs to perform. You want your oldest to be your baby's peer, not a surrogate parent.

DAY 228	DATE:
	38 days to go

The baby almost always settles into the mother's pelvis in a **head-down position**, because the head is the heaviest part of its body and is better accommodated in the bottom contour of the uterus than in the top.

If you give birth vaginally, your baby will leave your uterus through the cervix (the neck, or mouth, of the uterus). **When your cervix has dilated to 10 cm (4 inches), the baby can pass through.** Easy to say . . .

Consider This There are many forms of **intimate behavior** that help you and your partner feel emotionally close. You may find that intimacy feels more comfortable during a second pregnancy than during your first, since you already know you can produce a healthy baby.

Did You Know? **It's not uncommon for women to be dilated ⅓ to ¾ inch (1 or 2 cm) in the last month** but not to be in active labor or having many noticeable contractions.

For Your Health Stress, poor diet, and trauma can weaken the uterine muscle, bring on premature labor, and slow baby's brain development. **While you can't control what happens to you when tragedy strikes, you do have some control over how you react.** Be mindful of your pregnancy and your need for stability and nutrition. Enlist the help of other competent people to help you develop a plan of action. And in the meantime BREATHE . . . slowly 10 times, in through the nose and out through the mouth.

Parents are often so busy with the physical rearing of children that they miss the glory of parenthood, just as the grandeur of the trees is lost when raking leaves.
MARCELENE COX

DAY 229	DATE: *37 days to go*

A baby born at eight months will tend to lose considerably more weight than a full-term baby, because its digestive tract is still too immature for complete independence. **As a sort of safety precaution, the eight-month-old fetus stores nutrition from the mother against the possibility of an early birth.**

Between Weeks 16 and 40, 15 to 20 percent **more oxygen is captured by your lungs** from each volume of air you breathe.

Your practitioner will probably want to see you once a week until you go into labor. **Make sure you keep your appointments**, since it's important to monitor the frequency and duration of your contractions (if you have any), to determine if the baby has dropped, to assess swelling, weight gain, and blood pressure, and to test for protein and sugar in the urine.

Parenting Tip When you visit your practitioner, **write down any verbal instructions** he or she gives you. What seems clear in the office or clinic may become confusing by the time you get home. Bring a list of questions so you won't forget to ask. Don't hesitate to ask about anything that pertains to you or your baby.

Chart your waist size and weight here and on page 182.

WAIST SIZE   WEIGHT

....

DAY 230	DATE: *36 days to go*

By this time, your baby's skin looks pink and smooth because underlying deposits of fat have masked some of the redness of the capillaries. **Babies who will have darker skin later may have a pinkish cast now because their skin itself is still unpigmented.**

Your diaphragm is now elevated and tilted because of pressure from your enlarging uterus. **This change causes your rib cage to flare,** or open up slightly. The circumference of your chest may increase by almost 2½ inches (61 mm).

IMPORTANT: You may notice stronger and more frequent **Braxton-Hicks contractions**, some of which may even be painful. This is normal.

Parenting Tip When parents aren't around, **babies soothe themselves** with what are known as transitional objects—physical comforts that help ease a child's fear of separating from caregivers. For that reason, consider fostering such attachments early in your child's infancy by offering him or her a special blanket, plush toy, or a pacifier. A child's reliance on a transitional object is *not* a sign of insecurity—it's a coping mechanism.

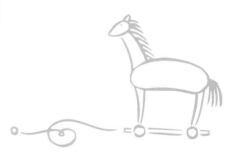

Nothing great was ever achieved without enthusiasm.

RALPH WALDO EMERSON

Easing the Transition from One Child to Two **Give your oldest some responsibility, if he or she wishes it.** Let your child be the baby's decision maker—selecting clothing, food items, and toys, when appropriate. If you make an offer, "Would you like to decide whether baby should have peas or green beans for lunch?" and he or she declines involvement, that should be fine, too.

DAY 231	DATE:
	35 days to go

Your baby's arms and legs are looking fuller and more rounded as more fat is deposited under the surface of the skin. Fat deposits increase from about 2 percent at mid-pregnancy to 12 to 15 percent at term. In a week or so, this fat will make up about 8 percent of your baby's body weight.

Iron transfer takes place at the placenta in one direction only: from you toward the baby. Five-sixths of the **iron stored in the baby's liver accumulates during the last trimester.** The stored iron will compensate in the baby's first four months out of the womb for inadequate amounts of iron in breast milk or formulas, so **make sure your iron intake is adequate.**

TIME TO REFLECT
What's one thing you want your baby to have that you didn't?

For Your Comfort During this last month, give yourself more opportunity to rest and relax. **Elevate your legs when you can and drink plenty of fluids.**

Parenting Tip You might not think infants really care which toys you choose to give them, but some toys can support the development of the child's early skills. For example, **first toys** might include those that are visually stimulating since the baby's eyes are learning to process form, line, shape, and color. Mobiles and high-contrast visual displays are good choices.

What do you want to be sure to remember?

(See page 180 for more space to write.)

Children don't have to be raised. They'll grow.
BUFFY SAINTE-MARIE

Week 34 Begins

DAY	DATE:
232	34 days to go

DAY	DATE:
233	33 days to go

Your baby has developed for 33 weeks. The operation of the umbilical cord has made it unnecessary for the **baby's slowly developing digestive system** to function much before birth. Even after birth, this system will still be functionally immature until the child is three or four years old.

Your basal metabolism rate increases 25 percent late in your pregnancy, so **your body is now 25 percent more efficient in converting stored nutrients to energy.** This increase is in response to the continuing demands of the baby on your system and the needs of your body's tissues.

Did You Know? From this point on, the "finishing period" of growth begins, during which **your baby prepares for its birth.**

Parenting Tip **To make crying less likely when you leave your baby with others,** try spending a few minutes with the child before leaving and not hurriedly rushing off. In addition, acquaint your firstborn with any new care providers or sleeping arrangements months before the birth of a sibling so your older child won't feel displaced or abandoned to a stranger once the baby comes.

During this finishing period of your baby's development, the fat being laid down under the surface of the skin helps the baby maintain an even body temperature and serves as a reserve that can be burned as energy. **Growth has slowed— perhaps to conserve energy for the birth process.**

A diet providing **2,400 calories** is generally still recommended at this point in your pregnancy to meet your energy requirements—unless you are physically inactive.

Did You Know? **You may actually begin to lose weight this month.** Weight loss of 2 to 3 lbs (908 to 1,362 g) is not uncommon as labor approaches and the baby's development is completed. **Don't try to diet** in these last weeks, however, even if you gained more weight than expected early in pregnancy.

IMPORTANT: Never leave a baby alone without **line-of-sight supervision.** Always pick up the baby and take him or her with you when you answer the phone or the door, even if that means interrupting a bath to do so. It only takes a second for an unsupervised baby to get into trouble.

Call it a clan, call it a network, call it a tribe, call it a family.
Whatever you call it, whoever you are, you need one.
JANE HOWARD

160

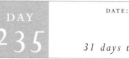

DAY 234

DATE:

32 days to go

Your baby's limbs are beginning to **dimple at the elbows and knees**, and **creases are forming around the wrists and neck** as fat deposit continues.

The circulatory requirements of your uterus have increased throughout your pregnancy as it enlarged and the baby and placenta developed. Now, near the end of your pregnancy, **one-sixth of your total blood volume is contained within the vessels of the uterus.**

IMPORTANT: You'll notice more **fluctuations in your energy level** this month. Fatigue is experienced by most pregnant women, but this month, you may find that fatigue alternates with periods of extra energy. Use your energy bursts wisely doing things you absolutely need to do and preparing for the birth and time after birth. Don't overdo it, though! You might need to conserve some of that energy for later.

Parenting Tip Before your baby begins to crawl, **cover all unused electrical outlets** with pronged plastic caps, available at hardware stores. Wind up excess lengths of plugged-in cords and fasten with rubber bands or twist-ties.

Easing the Transition from One Child to Two Understand your older child's inclination to want to act more like a baby once the baby arrives. **Be patient** with his or her interest in drinking from a bottle, using baby talk, wanting to sleep in the crib, even wanting to wear diapers. Mostly, he or she just wants to remember what it feels like to be so little. Make sure you show your "big baby" as much love and attention as your "new baby." At the same time, you can highlight all the things your oldest child can do that the baby cannot even attempt.

DAY 235

DATE:

31 days to go

Your baby's gums are now bumpy and may look at first like teeth are about to erupt. During labor, **the amniotic fluid** that surrounds the baby equalizes the pressure of the contractions, so one part of the baby's body is not pressed more than another. The amniotic fluid also prevents contractions from interfering with the blood flow from the placenta to the baby.

IMPORTANT: Keep in mind, your baby needs to eat even when you'd rather not. Several small meals a day are still best at this point for most women.

Parenting Tip **Devise different names to call grandparents** so your child can learn to tell them apart when people are speaking about them. Some grandparents choose their own names (Grandpa Joe or Grandma Jones) and some prefer nicknames.

Chart your waist size and weight here and on page 182.

WAIST SIZE   WEIGHT

No animal is so inexhaustible as an excited infant.

AMY LESLIE

DAY 236	DATE:
	30 days to go

By the time the baby is born, **the fully developed placenta** covers 15 to 30 percent of the space inside the uterus and will weigh 5½ lb—a little more than a large bag of flour. The placental tissue itself weighs a mere pound and a half, but it takes 4 lb of blood to keep it functional.

While your appetite and energy levels might fluctuate, **you'll probably notice more rather than less swelling** of your ankles, feet, hands, and face during these final weeks. About 40 percent of women have slight ankle swelling during the last twelve weeks of pregnancy. This swelling generally disappears with rest and is rarely present in the morning.

Any swelling you have that is associated with pain and does not disappear within 24 hours should be reported to your practitioner.

For Your Information Clear or pink-tinged mucous may be a sign that the **mucous plug**, which seals the opening of the uterus, has dislodged. This usually means that the cervix is beginning to dilate and that true labor may be days or even hours away.

Did You Know? Your **baby's digestive system**—from mouth to anus—will eventually be about 30 feet in length. At birth, its tiny stomach is about the size of a marble that expands to the size of a ping-pong ball after a few days of feedings.

What do you want to be sure to remember?

(See page 180 for more space to write.)

DAY 237	DATE:
	29 days to go

Within the next day or so, the percentage of **white fat** in your baby's body will have increased to 8 percent.

As your growing uterus puts pressure on your diaphragm, **your heart will become displaced** upward and to the left.

For Your Comfort **Leg cramps during sleep are common** late in pregnancy. Prevent cramps by avoiding fatigue and elevating your legs whenever possible.

Parenting Tip Your baby's nails will need to be trimmed so he or she won't scratch herself or others. A good time might be after a bath (nails are more pliable) or when the baby is nursing or asleep. Use nail clippers for babies or round-end scissors, and push the skin behind the nail down before you cut (you'll be upset if the skin bleeds).

A child's education should begin at least one hundred years before he is born.

OLIVER WENDELL HOLMES

Easing the Transition from One Child to Two Keep some together time with your older child intact after the baby arrives. Continue with the same traditions or routines (like the series of activities that leads up to bedtime) **so your older child feels a sense of continuity between his or her life before and after baby.**

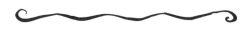

TIME TO REFLECT

"If my baby has _____, I'll be happy!"

Childbirth in Other Cultures In some cultures such as China, breast-feeding continues for up to six years.

Parenting Tip A healthy diet, good hygiene, and regular checkups are essential to your **baby's dental health.** Plaque forms on baby's teeth, too, and can be removed by rubbing a warm, wet gauze pad over the teeth and gums very gently—no toothpaste needed. The American Dental Association recommends that baby's first visit to the pediatric dentist occur around baby's first birthday or within six months after the appearance of the first tooth.

DAY	DATE:
2 3 8	*28 days to go*

It took eight weeks for your baby's body fat percentage to increase from 2 to 3 percent (Week 26) to 8 percent (Week 34). By the end of prenatal development, the baby's body fat percentage will stabilize at about 15 percent. This padding of fat will **help keep your baby warm and protected after birth.**

Your baby may become quite chubby **if you overeat** during this time. Even with normal weight gain, the baby now fits snugly in your womb and can only turn from side to side.

What do you want to be sure to remember?

(See page 180 for more space to write.)

How dear to this heart are the scenes of my childhood, / When fond recollection presents them to view!
SAMUEL WOODWORTH

Week 35 Begins

DAY 239	DATE:
	27 days to go

More than ninety percent of babies are **born within two weeks of their due dates**, either early or late. You and your baby are two weeks from that time frame now.

Your vaginal discharge will become heavier now and will contain more cervical mucous. The **discharge may be streaked** with recent (reddish or pink) or oxidized (brown) blood after intercourse or after a pelvic exam.

IMPORTANT: Watch for **symptoms of labor**, but don't be obsessed with them. Your baby's birthday could be just around the corner or it could be weeks away. **Take it one day at a time.**

Did You Know? **Your cervix is sensitive and blood-engorged right now**; bumping it may cause spotting.

Easing the Transition from One Child to Two **Immediately after birth, start building a positive relationship between your children** by pointing out how much the baby likes them. Help your other children to notice how baby smiles when they come near, how baby enjoys being near them, and how much baby likes the toys and kisses they offer. **It's difficult to dislike someone who likes you back.** If you must correct the older child, do it gently, offering much praise as you encourage any adjustments. An angry outburst or scolding may bring tears from both children and resentment from the firstborn.

DAY 240	DATE:
	26 days to go

The **flavors of all the foods and beverages** that the mother has eaten in the past few hours are transmitted to the fluid that surrounds the baby in the womb and to her breastmilk. For example, if you want baby to like broccoli later, eat it now! ☺

Fetal blood flows through **two umbilical arteries and one umbilical vein.** During late pregnancy, a soft blowing sound called "funic souffle" can be heard over the location of your baby's umbilical cord.

Bright red discharge or persistent spotting should be **reported to your practitioner** *immediately.*

IMPORTANT: While nearly 8 of 10 U.S. women breast-feed their newborns, less than 3 of 10 are still breast-feeding by 12 months. **Breast-feeding success** hinges on many factors, but the support of one's partner is crucial. Women whose partners supported breast-feeding gave more beneficial breast milk to their babies for a significantly longer period of time than women whose partners encouraged formula use.

Easing the Transition from One Child to Two Remember that for you, your partner, and your older child, developing a loving attachment to the baby involves **getting to know the baby**, and what his or her habits and preferences are, as baby gets to know each of you. Keep in mind, too, that having another baby may fit beautifully into your own plans, but may not have been on your older child's agenda at all.

The best inheritance a parent can give his children is a few minutes of his time each day.

O. A. BATTISTA

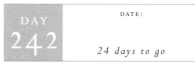

DAY 241	DATE:
	25 days to go

While the ossification process has been progressing steadily (cartilage turning into bone), **not all of your baby's bones will be ossified by birth.** This is an advantage for both of you. The baby's skeleton is more flexible when it contains more cartilage, making the passage through the narrow birth canal easier. Fewer hard bones mean fewer hard pokes during delivery!

The total weight of the **placenta** and supporting membranes by your due date is 1½ lb (680 g). The total weight of the **amniotic fluid** at term is 2 lb (907 g).

Take Note The **mucous plug** is often mistaken for **amniotic fluid**. The key difference is that the mucous plug is thick and looks like clear nasal mucous or mucous tinged with blood, while amniotic fluid is watery.

Parenting Tip **Always set a timer when you're cooking** with children around. Babies are distracting, and you can easily forget your food and cause a fire or ruin the food.

> *What do you want to be sure to remember?*

....

....

....

....

....

(See page 180 for more space to write.)

DAY 242	DATE:
	24 days to go

Your baby will now automatically turn toward a source of light. This is called the *orienting response* and permits your baby to practice being more aware of its environment.

There is generally little measured rise in blood pressure during a healthy pregnancy, in spite of the increased blood volume and increased demands on your heart. If anything, it will be highest during the last week of your pregnancy.

IMPORTANT: Basically, your baby will need a car safety seat, clothing, diapers, a place to sleep, food, and love once he or she is here. You can supply the love and the food (if you're breast-feeding), but **do you have everything else you'll need for the first couple of weeks after the birth?**

Parenting Tip The availability of **powdered breast milk** would certainly give formula makers a competitive challenge. But what about its benefit to the baby? The antibody value of powdered milk would be lost in processing in the same way that microwaving frozen breast milk destroys immune benefits. Other nutrients would be compromised by processing, and the composition of the milk wouldn't change as the baby's growth needs changed. In addition, the milk couldn't be benefited by enriching the diet of the mother. **But the question remains:** Would powdered breast milk be better for baby overall than powdered formula?

> *Always be nice to your children because they are the ones who will choose your rest home.*
> PHYLLIS DILLER

DAY 243

DATE:

23 days to go

The round, plump look of the typical new-born is normal and healthy. Your baby's **birth weight is unrelated to his or her likelihood of later obesity.**

Braxton-Hicks contractions—false labor pains—are believed to facilitate circulation to and through the placenta by stimulating the movement of the blood.

For Your Comfort **It's important to plan ahead**, so you can relax as much as possible before and during delivery, knowing everything has been taken care of. If you have a freezer, you and your partner might begin stocking it with easy-to-prepare foods.

IMPORTANT: Keep in mind that the challenges of the time right after the baby's birth might be intensified by **mood swings** called the "baby blues." If you had postpartum blues the first time, you remember that unexplained crying, feeling out of control, irritability, lack of energy (even after sleeping), problems sleeping, and depression are involved. If you didn't have the baby blues with your first birth, expect them with your second, since the odds are 50/50 with second and third babies. If you experienced any depression before or during your pregnancy, the likelihood of baby blues is increased. For most women, these feelings resolve within two weeks, especially with good physical care, emotional support, and help taking care of the baby. **If the symptoms don't go away after two to three weeks, if the feelings of inadequacy worsen, if they prevent you from taking care of yourself or the baby, or if they involve thoughts about hurting the baby, let your practitioner know right away.**

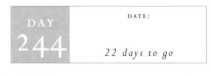

Tell your practitioner about any of these kinds of feelings as soon as you become aware of them.

DAY 244

DATE:

22 days to go

The baby maintains a temperature that is **about 3.2°F above the mother's temperature.**

Because the baby's quarters are so cramped at this point, when he or she moves, the contours of his or her **arms and legs make moving bulges on your abdomen.** It should be fairly easy for you to identify the baby's arms and legs, but you may confuse the head with the buttocks through the stretched skin of your abdomen.

Did You Know? You will notice that for several weeks after birth, **your baby will maintain the fetal position** it was forced to assume in the uterus, because its muscles are used to it.

IMPORTANT: Everybody needs help with a new baby. Start arranging for that help now. For example, perhaps a friend could help by bringing lunch by for several days after the birth. If the people you know are inclined to give gifts, perhaps you could suggest they give the gift of assistance (bringing over nutritious meals, staying with the baby in the afternoon so you can take a nap, cleaning up a bit, etc.). On the other hand, you may be too tired for company!

Chart your waist size and weight here and on page 182.

WAIST SIZE   WEIGHT

Children are the wisdom of the nation.
LIBERIAN PROVERB

DAY **245**	DATE: *21 days to go*

This date ends Week 35 of your baby's development. From this point forward, **your baby's growth will be much slower until birth, except for fat production.** In these last two weeks, the average baby gains about 14 g of fat, roughly the equivalent of 1¼ tablespoons of butter (which is 100 percent fat).

As you approach delivery, the amniotic sac (bag of waters) may break. Generally, it's more of a trickle than a gush. If you're concerned about fluid leakage when you're not at home, wear a pad or panty liner to absorb the moisture. Amniotic fluid has its own distinct odor and can easily be distinguished from urine.

Contact your practitioner if you think you're leaking amniotic fluid.

Ready to Breast-Feed You'll have to consume 400–500 extra calories per day, **mostly in the form of complex carbohydrates and protein**, while breast-feeding to keep your energy up. But don't worry, you'll be hungry all the time!

TIME TO REFLECT
What does your pregnancy mean to your family?

What do you want to be sure to remember?

(See page 180 for more space to write.)

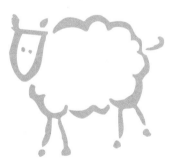

You have to ask children and birds how cherries and strawberries taste.

J. W. GOETHE

LMP Week 38

<table>
<tr><td>DAY
246</td><td>DATE:

20 days to go</td></tr>
</table>

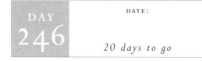

Your baby's intestines are accumulating considerable meconium, a dark-green mixture of used cells and waste products from the baby's liver, pancreas, and gall bladder.

You've probably discussed **the difference between false labor and true labor** with your practitioner. The main points will be reviewed over the next several journal days to keep them fresh in your mind.

FALSE vs. TRUE LABOR: With Braxton-Hicks, or false labor, contractions, the pain begins in your lower abdomen. The contractions that accompany **true labor begin in your lower back and the pain spreads to your lower abdomen.**

Childbirth in Other Cultures In the Yucatán, other women beside the midwife and woman's mother may be called in to give mental and physical support during a difficult labor. Traditionally, these women encourage her, sometimes scold her, always let her know she is not alone, and tell her that the business of giving birth will soon be done, because they have all experienced what she is going through.

Parenting Tip **Apply a cold pack for bumps and bruises in the first 24 hours** after injury by pressing lightly for 20 minutes. Frozen fruit bars can be useful in soothing bumped lips; a bag of frozen vegetables works well as a flexible compress. You may prefer using purchased compresses that can be refrozen and reused.

<table>
<tr><td>DAY
247</td><td>DATE:

19 days to go</td></tr>
</table>

The meconium in your baby's intestines will be eliminated shortly after birth, but it sometimes can be eliminated before, if the birth is delayed too long. In the latter case, this dark-green material will be present at birth in the amniotic fluid.

By today, your baby's toenails have reached the ends of the toes. As a point of interest, the fingernails and toenails actually begin to form on the palm of the hand and sole of the foot and then migrate to their final positions at the end of each digit.

IMPORTANT: If you feel like you have **extra energy, save it for your labor**—don't weed your entire garden or clean out all your closets!

Parenting Tip **Never leave plastic bags where children can find them.** Even small pieces of plastic can cause children to suffocate. Get in the habit of knotting all plastic bags before recycling them. Better yet, use repeat-use bags and avoid the accumulation of plastic altogether.

What do you want to be sure to remember?

(See page 180 for more space to write.)

The soul is healed by being with children.

FYODOR DOSTOEVSKY

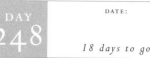

DAY
248

DATE:

18 days to go

Within the next three days, **the circumference of your baby's head will roughly match the circumference of his or her shoulders and hips.** After this time, the abdomen may be greater than the head.

FALSE vs. TRUE LABOR: The contractions of **true labor become progressively stronger and more painful as time passes and aren't interrupted by changing one's position.**

Childbirth in Other Cultures In the Mayan culture, a midwife traditionally gives a woman a special massage 20 days after she gives birth. This massage marks the end of the postpartum period.

Parenting Tip **If your baby feels warm** when you press your lips to his or her forehead, check first to make sure baby isn't overdressed or overwrapped. If the baby isn't feeling well and you want to take his or her temperature, a rectal thermometer with some lubricant inserted about an inch is most accurate. Your pediatrician will tell you that if your baby is three months old or younger and registers a rectal temperature of 100.4°F (38°C), call him or her *immediately*.

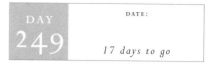

DAY
249

DATE:

17 days to go

As you might expect, the baby's limbs are bent and drawn even closer to his or her body and his or her hands are tightly fisted. Because of the space limitations in the uterus now, **the movements of your baby are quite restricted.**

FALSE vs. TRUE LABOR: When **timing contractions** (your practitioner will have you look for contractions a certain number of minutes apart), don't expect perfect, even intervals (i.e., contraction, 6 minutes/3 seconds, contraction, 6 minutes/3 seconds, etc.). If, for example, you are supposed to call your practitioner when your contractions are four minutes apart, expect them to be about four minutes apart rather than exactly four minutes apart.

Childbirth in Other Cultures When a traditional Comanche woman is in labor, she goes to a clearing a short distance from her camp where three four-foot stakes are set in the ground 10 feet apart. She walks while she labors, and, during each contraction, she kneels down near a stake, grasping it on a level with her head. She is assisted by a female relative.

Parenting Tip When you pick your newborn up, be sure to **place one hand under the baby's neck** to support his or her head and **the other hand under his or her back and bottom** to support his or her lower half. **Head support is particularly important**—the baby will have no control over it at all until he or she is about four weeks old.

*Parents: People who spend half their time wondering how their children will turn out,
and the rest of the time when they will turn in.*

ELEANOR GRAHAM VANCE

DAY	DATE:
250	*16 days to go*

In about another week, your baby's foot will be slightly longer than the length of his or her thigh. Take a look at your own thigh to see how big that is relative to the size of your feet. Such **odd proportions** will change somewhat after birth.

FALSE vs. TRUE LABOR: **If you stand or walk when you're having a contraction, the force of gravity will make the contractions more efficient and will reduce the time of labor.** By the end of pregnancy, the muscle cells of the vagina are enlarged and there is less supportive connective tissue. Thus, the vaginal walls have become sufficiently relaxed to permit the passage of the baby during birth.

Childbirth in Other Cultures Among the Santa Maria Indians of Guatemala, it is the custom for the midwife, both grandmothers, the husband, and sometimes the father-in-law to attend the birth.

Parenting Tip **Baby wipes** are versatile! You can also use them to **1.** Clean dirt and blood off scrapes and bruises. **2.** Remove makeup. **3.** Clean your hands after pumping gas. **4.** Soothe sunburns. **5.** Wipe down restroom surfaces. **6.** Substitute for toilet paper. Make sure the baby wipes are moistened with natural substances and are disposed of responsibly.

DAY	DATE:
251	*15 days to go*

If your baby is a girl, during the last three or so days the outer lips (labia) of the vulva have formed over the smaller inner lips underneath.

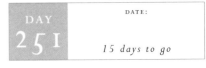

Frequent urination can help labor progress: A full bladder will push against the uterus, causing discomfort.

Childbirth in Other Cultures The Mayan woman who sits behind the laboring mother and supports her arms and body is called the "head helper." She supports the mother's weight and shadows the mother's pushing and breathing during contractions.

Parenting Tip When you're out of the house with the baby, you might want to use a sling or backpack to hold your wallet, cell phone, and other necessities **so you'll have one less thing to carry.**

Consider This You'll want to look into clean, natural formula and organic foods for **infants and toddlers.** Milk by-products used to make organic formulas come from cows that were not given growth hormones or antibiotics and that eat pesticide-free feed. **Organic products reduce your baby's level of exposure to harmful chemicals.**

Chart your waist size and weight here and on page 182.

WAIST SIZE   WEIGHT

Every baby born into the world is a finer one than the last.
CHARLES DICKENS

DAY 252	DATE:
	14 days to go

At this point in development, the **average baby** weighs about 6⅓ lb (2,900 g) and measures almost 13½ inches (34 cm). Professional male basketball players generally have big feet because they are so tall. Your baby could be cradled in one of their size 18 shoes (a new one, of course!).

Use relaxation exercises, such as breathing in through your nose and out through your mouth, to help **ease the pain of contractions.**

Childbirth in Other Cultures A number of tribes lubricate a laboring woman's birth canal with saps or oils to make the delivery easier.

Ready to Breast-Feed **Breast-feeding is an intense experience, especially during the first month.** You are feeding your baby every two to three hours around the clock. You are probably eating and sleeping when the baby does, so you're tired. And you're also trying to use your breast pump to stimulate your production. And even though you know this is what you need and want to do, at times you can feel like one big worn-out mammary gland. **But take heart.** Over time, your baby will start to consolidate sleep time into bigger chunks and begin to sleep more at night than during the day. And slowly, your days will stop merging together. This is the time when partners and moms and grandmothers and aunts and sisters and best friends do heroic things for you, and you're truly grateful.

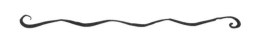

TIME TO REFLECT

What's one thing you can do to take even better care of yourself?

What do you want to be sure to remember?

(See page 180 for more space to write.)

By the time we realize our parents may have been right, we usually have children who think we're wrong.
ANONYMOUS

LMP Week 39

DAY 253	DATE:
	13 days to go

Contrary to popular understanding, human development before birth actually **requires nine and a half lunar months, not nine.** These last two weeks are part of that additional period.

FALSE vs. TRUE LABOR: The contractions of **true labor may be accompanied by diarrhea.**

Childbirth in Other Cultures If a laboring woman is tiring or progress is slowing, many cultures know to massage or pinch the woman's nipples so that oxytocin will be released into her system. This is the same substance that is used in synthetic form in the United States and other Western cultures to induce labor.

Parenting Tip When you use **skin-care products** on your face and body, a small amount of the product is absorbed by your skin and enters your system and, ultimately, the baby's. **Check with your health-care provider about using safer skin-care products while you're pregnant.**

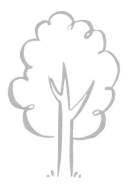

DAY 254	DATE:
	12 days to go

Over the next couple of days, your baby's lungs will begin to increase their production of a surfactant, a thick substance which **keeps the air sacs in the lungs open.**

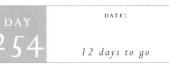 Your uterus is highly muscular and weighs 2½ lb (1,134 g) now that the baby is fully developed. **During a contraction, the uterus feels hard to the touch.**

Chart your waist size and weight here and on page 182.

WAIST SIZE   WEIGHT

IMPORTANT: Be prepared to call your practitioner when signs indicate that you're ready to go to the hospital or birth center or ready to begin the process of home birth. Don't worry about the time of day. **People who attend births expect to be called at all hours!**

Ready to Breast-Feed You can be informed, well supplied, organized, diligent, and encouraged and *still* have problems breast-feeding. You may develop a painful infection in your breast or along your C-section incision; your baby may have a weak sucking reflex because she's premature; you may become sick with a cold or the flu or need to be hospitalized; there may be a crisis that needs your attention. And if that's not enough, any stress you experience can make it even more difficult to breast-feed because you can't relax and let the milk flow. **Definitely stay with it and give breast-feeding your very best effort.** But if you've tried as hard as you can and exhausted every resource, it's okay. Now for Plan B . . .

Boy: A noise with some dirt on it.

SAMUEL TAYLOR COLERIDGE

172

DAY 255	DATE:
	11 days to go

From about this point on, your baby will gain about ½ oz (14 g) of fat each day it stays in your uterus. Three U.S. quarters weigh about ½ oz.

The muscles at the top of your uterus apply **a force comparable to a weight of 55 lb (24.5 kg) during each contraction.** This shows how much force must be applied to resistant muscles to open the cervix and push the baby out of the uterus during birth!

IMPORTANT: Keep your list of emergency phone numbers in a convenient place. **If you're in labor and can't get to the hospital, birthing center, or in touch with your midwife, dial 911** or the emergency number for your area. Unlock your door, lie down, and pant to avoid pushing until help arrives. Labor can take many hours, however, so don't panic if you must wait a little while for assistance.

Parenting Tip **Make sure your children will be well cared for while you are giving birth.** Even if you will be at home, you can't attend to their needs during labor and delivery (and even for a while afterward). Arrange for someone to be there to watch your children.

DAY 256	DATE:
	10 days to go

The lanugo (downy hair that once covered your baby's body) is disappearing. **If any of the lanugo remains by birth, it will be found on the baby's shoulders, forehead, and neck.**

FALSE vs. TRUE LABOR: You might be interested in **other women's descriptions of the experience of true labor.** Many women compare the contractions of true labor to waves: gathering, rising, breaking, falling. **The pressure builds in the uterine muscles and reaches a peak that lasts 30 to 50 seconds or so.** Then the pressure disappears rapidly. When it's over, you feel nothing until the next contraction. To some, the gripping sensation of the contraction feels like bad menstrual cramps or intestinal cramps. Most women report that persistent backache accompanies the contractions. **Labor is a well-named phenomenon. It's the work that you will do to give birth to your baby. Although the work is difficult, few jobs are as rewarding or satisfying.**

Childbirth in Other Cultures Many cultures believe that the placenta needs to be treated in a special way because it is part of the baby's soul.

For Your Comfort **Citrus drops or herbal throat drops** are nice to have on hand during labor to help keep your mouth from drying.

The toughest thing about raising kids is convincing them that you have seniority.
ANONYMOUS

DAY 257	DATE:
	9 days to go

In a few days, your baby's fingernails will extend beyond his or her fingertips. Your newborn may have no functioning tear ducts for a couple of weeks. **The first cries are almost always tearless ones.**

There are many reasons why **you might have more difficulty sleeping from now on.** The baby may be much more active, you may be experiencing periodic contractions, and you're probably anxious and anticipating the birth. All of this is very predictable and common.

IMPORTANT: Try to **relax** and be as comfortable as you can. **Rest** whenever you feel tired.

Parenting Tip **Some parents might want to involve existing siblings in the birth event.** Home birth and birthing centers can accommodate children. The age and personality of each individual child is an important consideration. Not all children will react positively to childbirth. Some children might be fascinated by all the activity; some might be scared; some might be bored and restless. Make sure you have someone on hand to take care of the needs of the attending children. If the siblings are hungry or tired or want to do something else, this caretaking adult can take over and see that their needs are met in a safe and timely way.

DAY 258	DATE:
	8 days to go

The **average length of a newborn's umbilical cord** is 2 ft (610 mm), but the cord can vary from 5 inches (127 mm) to almost 4 ft (1,219 mm) long. By the time of birth, the cord is capable of transmitting about 300 quarts (284 liters) of fluid per day—almost 75 gallons of milk!

When the baby settles deep into your pelvis, **you may feel clumsy and off-balance.** That's because your center of gravity has shifted as the baby changed its position.

Childbirth in Other Cultures In many nonindustrial cultures, a mother and newborn baby stay in their own hut, where they rest and recuperate without distraction, away from the other members of their group.

Parenting Tip If you haven't already done so, **think about investing in a system that can record and store still pictures and real-time video**—one that's reliable, easy to use, there when you need it, makes it easy to share pictures, and, of course, priced within your budget. You can never have too many pictures of your baby!

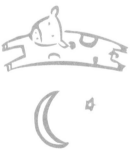

Hit a child and quarrel with its mother.
NIGERIAN PROVERB

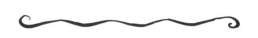

DAY 259	DATE:
	7 days to go

The color of your baby's skin is begin-ning to change from reddish or pinkish to white or bluish pink (even in babies with dark pigmentation). Changes in your baby's skin color are due to the growing thickness of the fatty layer under the skin's surface. Earlier in development, the skin was so transparent and layered with so little fat that if you could have seen your baby, you would have seen its organs through its skin. Now, the growing layer of fat gives your baby's skin an opaque quality and masks the color of the muscles and circulating blood cells.

Week 37 draws to a close. You may notice more of **a change in the way you walk**, since your balance is being thrown off by your enlarged uterus and the shifting position of the baby.

Childbirth in Other Cultures Tribal societies tend to have a fairly long transition period after birth, during which the baby is nursed and cared for by the mother, sleeps with the mother, and is attended to quickly when it cries. The more industrialized a society is, the shorter the transition period. Scandinavian coun-tries, like Sweden and Denmark, are the exception. They offer generous parental leaves to their citizens.

Parenting Tip During its first year, **take a picture of your baby each month at about the same time** (first week, third week, on the 15th, etc.). If the picture is taken in the same pose or by the same furniture, it will be easier to see the dramatic changes in the baby's growth. After the first year, take photo records at least twice a year.

TIME TO REFLECT

What's the most important skill you can practice as a parent?

What do you want to be sure to remember?

(See page 180 for more space to write.)

We've had bad luck with our kids—they've all grown up.
CHRISTOPHER MORLEY

Week 38 Begins

DAY 260	DATE:
	6 days to go

Your baby's skull is not yet fully solid. It is made up of five large bony plates that are separated and will be pushed together, or overlapped during birth.

During these last few weeks in the womb, the **baby continues to receive one of the most important ingredients for survival from your blood, from the placenta, and also from the amniotic fluid** (which is swallowed periodically): disease-combating antibodies that will provide an immunity to a wide range of illnesses.

For Your Health **Don't push yourself right now.** Just rest, eat well, and nurture yourself as the baby's birthday approaches.

Did You Know? **The base of the baby's skull is the first part of the head to form into bone.** At 20 weeks, the plates that cover the forehead, temples, and top and back of the skull are all made of cartilage.

Chart your waist size and weight here and on page 182.

WAIST SIZE   WEIGHT

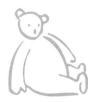

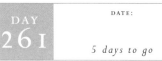

DAY 261	DATE:
	5 days to go

Over the next three days, **the last of the vernix** (the creamy protective substance on the surface of your baby's skin) will begin to disappear. The spaces between the bony plates of your baby's skull are called **fontanels**, which means "little fountains," because the pulse of your baby's bloodstream can be easily felt by touching them. The best known of the fontanels is the "**soft spot**" on the top of baby's head. **Don't worry if your baby's head becomes molded or elongated** during the birth process. It will return to its normal, rounded shape in a few days. The molding is a safety precaution—the bones of the skull carefully slide over one another to reduce the skull's diameter, so the pressure of the contractions and tight fit through the mother's pelvis doesn't damage the baby's brain.

Most babies drop into a headfirst, face-down position in their mother's pelvis. In some cases, the baby is in a headfirst, face-up position, so the back of its head presses against the mother's tailbone or spine. This produces the phenomenon called **back labor.** The pain of back labor is especially intense and doesn't seem to let up, even between contractions.

For Your Health From now until the baby is born, **continue walking for exercise and practice your breathing and relaxation exercises.** If your back is particularly sore, you might try to relieve some of the pain by gently stretching those muscles. When you begin having contractions, walking and controlled breathing will both help you through them.

Happy is he that is happy in his children.

THOMAS FULLER

Parenting Tip If you have to travel by plane, carry a small infant in a front pack so you can have your arms free. **Nurse your baby or give it a bottle or a pacifier during takeoff and landing to reduce the pressure in its ears.**

DAY 262	DATE:
	4 days to go

Over the next three days, **your baby's chest will become more prominent.** The breasts of boy and girl babies may become swollen because of the female sex hormone estrogen transferred from the mother's system. **The baby's abdomen will be big and round** at birth because of the liver's important role in producing red blood cells.

A kick from the womb during this stage of pregnancy can almost knock a book off your lap!

For Your Comfort If holidays or other celebrations that you actively plan or participate in are approaching, **shift responsibilities to other family members or friends for right now.** You need to have all pressures taken off so you can concentrate on the birth of your baby.

Parenting Tip Your baby has gotten used to feeling snug and secure in your uterus and, after birth, may sleep better and feel more comfortable if the pre-birth environment is duplicated. **Try swaddling** the baby snugly in a thin receiving blanket. **The safest sleeping position for infants under the age of one is lying on their backs; they can also be propped up on one side or the other, but** *never* **on their stomachs.**

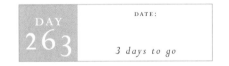

What do you want to be sure to remember?

(See page 180 for more space to write.)

DAY 263	DATE:
	3 days to go

If any of the vernix (the creamy protective substance on the surface of your baby's skin) remains until birth, it is usually found only on your baby's back. **As the vernix sloughs off the baby's skin, the amniotic fluid may change from clear and straw-colored to milky.** By about this time, baby is surrounded by 3 to 4½ cups (700 to 1,000 ml) of amniotic fluid.

It is the fortune commonly of knavish children to have the loving'st mothers.
THOMAS MIDDLETON

At this point, you might **consider taking a parenting class or doing some reading on child development, even if you are an experienced mom.** Such coursework can't hurt and may help you connect with your baby and with other mothers and professionals who can provide information and support. In addition, there are *always* new findings to review and new insights to consider about labor, delivery, child development, and parenting.

Childbirth in Other Cultures In the Myanmar Republic (also known as Burma), new mothers are traditionally fed a soup made with fish, plants, and fruit.

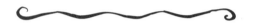

TIME TO REFLECT
Almost there! Would you do it all again?

....

....

....

....

....

of the lungs is *not* the inflation of empty organs but the rapid replacement of the fluid in the lungs by air. Pressure on the baby's chest during birth does help clear some fluid, however, as does the practitioner's active suctioning of baby's mouth and nose.

Each of your breasts gains about 1½ lb (672 g) during pregnancy in preparation for nursing. Time to go bra shopping!

Did You Know? Because **breast-feeding is a learned skill and not an instinct,** make sure you have lined up support from experienced nursing mothers or lactation specialists. You may need to call on them for advice or encouragement after the baby is born.

Parenting Tip While the baby is in your uterus, its world sounds watery and sloshy. **After baby is born, machines can duplicate those uterine sounds,** or play the sound of a running river, rain, a waterfall, or other water sounds, which may be soothing and help lull your baby to sleep.

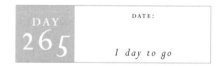

	DATE:
DAY **265**	*1 day to go*

By this time, about 15 percent of the baby's body is **fat.** About 80 percent of this fat is located directly under the surface of your baby's **skin,** while the other 20 percent is found on **organs and muscle tissue.**

Your weight gain has probably slowed or even reversed itself in the past two weeks or so.

For Your Information Relative to the size of the head, **your baby's face will look small at birth** because of the small size of the jaws, absence of nasal sinuses, and underdevelopment of the facial bones.

	DATE:
DAY **264**	*2 days to go*

The first breaths your baby takes are the hardest. It has been calculated that the first breathing-in requires five times the effort of an ordinary breath, because fluid must be pushed out of the lungs before the air drawn in can expand the thousands of tiny air sacs in the lungs. It is an effort that can be compared to clearing a snorkel tube that has gotten water in it. In this way, aeration

Give a little love to a child, and you get a great deal back.
JOHN RUSKIN

Increases in the size of the **nasal sinuses** (after age three or four) alter the shape of your baby's face and add resonance to the voice.

Did You Know? After birth, your baby's hair will grow at a rate of about ½ **inch (13 mm) a month!**

Ready to Breast-Feed You may enjoy your breast-feeding experience more if you get a break from time to time. **You can pump and store some milk**, then someone else can feed baby while you go out to lunch, get a massage, a pedicure, or hit the gym. Instead of conventional shower gifts, ask your friends to give you "Get Out of the House Free" cards that you can turn in to them for a little R & R when you need it.

DAY 266	DATE: *Due date*

Today is your baby's estimated due date. **Your baby is considered fully developed at this point.** If born today, your baby will weigh about 7½ lb (3,400 g) and measure about 14 inches (360 mm) **crown to rump**. Of course, baby's length at birth will be measured from head to toe and will be closer to 19 to 20 inches (50 cm). At birth, the average boy is slightly longer and heavier than the average girl. The chest is prominent in both sexes.

As you get to this point, you will find that you have more and more trouble sleeping and getting around. It's difficult to find any comfortable position, and if the baby is moving frequently or if you are experiencing Braxton-Hicks contractions, you may not be able to sleep even when you are comfortable. Try to relax and rest when you can. **It's difficult to be on any type of routine now.**

Childbirth in Other Cultures In cultures where new mothers spend more solitary time with their babies, births tend to be spaced fairly far apart. In cultures where women are given less transition time after the birth and return to work and household chores sooner, births tend to be more closely spaced.

Parenting Tip Tip: In the United States, the toll-free number for the **American Association of Poison Control Centers (AAPCC) is 1-800-222-1222.** Put the number on speed dial. Anything your baby might touch, ingest, or encounter that can make him or her sick can be considered a poison. These items include drugs/medicines, food and beverages, household products, environmental toxins, and animal and insect bites and stings. Your baby doesn't have to have symptoms for you to call. For example, a parent might call and say, "I just found my 10-month-old with a capsule from a medicine bottle that absorbs moisture. I don't know if she had it in her mouth, or bit part of it. All I know is that she had in her hand and I need to know what to do." The Center staff offer free, confidential, nonjudgmental, 24-hour medical advice. Almost every parent finds themselves making a call like this at some point in their child's life. **Welcome to the club!**

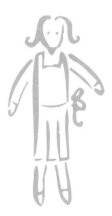

We can't give our children the future, strive though we may to make it secure. But we can give them the present.
KATHLEEN NORRIS

What do you want to remember about your
Ninth (and last!) Month?

(See pages 187 to 192 for entering labor and delivery details.)

Just Look at How You've Grown!

Record your waist size and weight here for easy comparisons. There are also places for you to record additional measurements, if you wish.

PAGE	DATE	WAIST SIZE	WEIGHT
10			

PAGE	DATE	WAIST SIZE	WEIGHT
16			

PAGE	DATE	WAIST SIZE	WEIGHT
20			

PAGE	DATE	WAIST SIZE	WEIGHT
24			

PAGE	DATE	WAIST SIZE	WEIGHT
30			

PAGE	DATE	WAIST SIZE	WEIGHT
38			

PAGE	DATE	WAIST SIZE	WEIGHT
42			

PAGE	DATE	WAIST SIZE	WEIGHT
46			

PAGE	DATE	WAIST SIZE	WEIGHT
53			

PAGE	DATE	WAIST SIZE	WEIGHT
56			

PAGE	DATE	WAIST SIZE	WEIGHT
61			

PAGE	DATE	WAIST SIZE	WEIGHT
65			

PAGE	DATE	WAIST SIZE	WEIGHT
69			

PAGE	DATE	WAIST SIZE	WEIGHT
74			

PAGE	DATE	WAIST SIZE	WEIGHT
78			

PAGE	DATE	WAIST SIZE	WEIGHT
82			

PAGE	DATE	WAIST SIZE	WEIGHT
87			

PAGE	DATE	WAIST SIZE	WEIGHT
93			

PAGE	DATE	WAIST SIZE	WEIGHT
96			

PAGE	DATE	WAIST SIZE	WEIGHT
99			

PAGE	DATE	WAIST SIZE	WEIGHT
148			

PAGE	DATE	WAIST SIZE	WEIGHT
106			

PAGE	DATE	WAIST SIZE	WEIGHT
153			

PAGE	DATE	WAIST SIZE	WEIGHT
109			

PAGE	DATE	WAIST SIZE	WEIGHT
158			

PAGE	DATE	WAIST SIZE	WEIGHT
113			

PAGE	DATE	WAIST SIZE	WEIGHT
161			

PAGE	DATE	WAIST SIZE	WEIGHT
117			

PAGE	DATE	WAIST SIZE	WEIGHT
166			

PAGE	DATE	WAIST SIZE	WEIGHT
122			

PAGE	DATE	WAIST SIZE	WEIGHT
170			

PAGE	DATE	WAIST SIZE	WEIGHT
127			

PAGE	DATE	WAIST SIZE	WEIGHT
172			

PAGE	DATE	WAIST SIZE	WEIGHT
130			

PAGE	DATE	WAIST SIZE	WEIGHT
176			

PAGE	DATE	WAIST SIZE	WEIGHT
133			

PAGE	DATE	WAIST SIZE	WEIGHT
183			

PAGE	DATE	WAIST SIZE	WEIGHT
141			

PAGE	DATE	WAIST SIZE	WEIGHT
184			

PAGE	DATE	WAIST SIZE	WEIGHT
144			

PAGE	DATE	WAIST SIZE	WEIGHT
186			

Full Term Plus 1

Chart your waist size and weight here and on page 182.

WAIST SIZE   WEIGHT

If your baby's expected date of delivery came and went, **don't worry**—you're not going to be pregnant forever. Remember that **the due date was just an estimate**, and while the baby's prenatal development has been completed, every baby is different and will be born in its own time.

Full Term Plus 2

Scientists are still not exactly sure what triggers the process of labor. It might involve the weight and size of the fetus putting pressure on the cervix, as well as the biochemical balance of your body—especially since the uterus becomes more and more sensitive to certain enzymes and hormones as pregnancy continues. **Nipple stimulation and male semen can encourage uterine contractions. Walking doesn't seem to help.**

Full Term Plus 3

If you're feeling **a little impatient** to give birth, that's okay. It's normal to want to get on with the process, even though you know it will be difficult and somewhat painful. Sometimes, however, impatience leads to feeling anxious and upset. It's important to stay as calm and composed as you can. Emotional distress is not going to be productive; in fact, it's going to tax your energy reserves. Try to distract yourself from negative emotions if you can't be positive and hopeful. Just hold on. You can do it.

Full Term Plus 4

So what's going on now that you and your baby are in this holding pattern? The baby is quite prepared for life outside the womb. Its lungs are still manufacturing large quantities of surfactant, in order to keep the air sacs of the lungs open. In general, your baby just continues to grow. Its hair gets longer, the nails grow, and it puts on more weight. If your baby is growing so large that a vaginal birth would be difficult, your practitioner may suggest that your labor be induced or a C-section performed.

Full Term Plus 5

You can't be pregnant forever. The placenta is an extremely functional organ, but it's a temporary one. It can sustain a normal human pregnancy, but it begins to break down in the weeks that follow the due date. Your practitioner will monitor placental functioning. Helping the placenta stay healthy involves the same activities on your part as keeping your developing baby healthy.

Well . . . Any thoughts? Feelings? Wishes?

All the time we wondered and wondered
who is this person coming / growing / turning / floating / swimming deep, deep inside.
CRESCENT DRAGONWAGON

Full Term Plus 6

While humans don't have the shortest pregnancies compared to other species, we certainly don't have the longest either. The Asiatic elephant (the one with the small ears) carries its babies for 20 to 23 months. If humans had 23-month pregnancies, you wouldn't even be halfway yet! The shortest pregnancies of mammals are found among opossums and an Australian animal called the eastern native cat. They carry their young for only 8 to 13 days before giving birth. **Imagine having the ability to give birth two or three times a month rather than just once a year!**

Full Term Plus 7

Chart your waist size and weight here and on page 182.

WAIST SIZE   WEIGHT

Take care to **write down the details of your baby's birth** so your child can learn the story of his or her birthday. Do you know the story of your own birth? If you do, write it down, and plan to relate it to your child when he or she's old enough, so your child can compare your births. If you don't know the details of your birth, ask your mother or someone else who would know.

Full Term Plus 8

Even though your baby is now one week past due, you're still well within the norm. In fact, 85 percent of all births are within two weeks of the estimated delivery date, either before or after. You and your baby just happen to be after, that's all. **As long as your practitioner is satisfied with your health and your baby's, there's nothing to worry about.**

Full Term Plus 9

If you don't already know the sex of your baby, you might want to make your prediction now. Do you think girls or boys run in certain families? Do you have both boy and girl names picked out? What prompted you to select those names? As you amuse yourself with these exercises, **remember that your baby's gender is not the most important thing about them. How your baby is doing is far more important.** Continue to take steps to eat well, stay hydrated, and rest so you can have a healthy baby.

So . . . how are you doing?

If children grew up according to early indications, we should have nothing but geniuses.

J. W. GOETHE

Full Term Plus 10

If you already have children at home, spend some time planning how you will integrate this new little sister or brother into the existing family. The older your child is, the more aware he or she will be of your pregnancy and of your preparations for the new baby. **Every son and daughter needs attention, their own space, and time to spend with family members as they choose.** Furthermore, most children don't like change, so if your son or daughter has to transition out of the crib and into a toddler bed to make room for baby, make the change slowly and begin preparations early enough to have him or her well settled. If they don't want to make the transition you have in mind, don't force or shame them into compliance; instead, come up with a new plan. When the time is right, teach your older children how to care for, play with, lift, hug, and feed the baby, and then let them decide what role they will play. If they want to be a caregiver, fine. If they don't, that should be fine, too. Try to be patient and understand everyone's needs.

Full Term Plus 11

Where will your new baby sleep? In most of the world's cultures, babies and young children sleep in the same bed as their parents. In the United States, however, such arrangements are discouraged for babies under the age of one year who have parents who are deep sleepers, are under the influence of alcohol or other drugs, or are extremely tired. Having baby sleep close by, however, offers easy access to the child and easy breast-feeding. Some of the disadvantages of baby sleeping close by involve parents who are light sleepers, adjustments for intimacy, and the eventual weaning of the child to their own room. Some parents worry that if their baby is in another room, they won't hear it. Unless the parent is a very deep sleeper, he or she will learn to respond to the sound of the baby's cry. **You'll have to decide what arrangement best serves your needs while keeping your baby safe.**

Hmm . . . Any news?

(See pages 187 to 192 for entering labor and delivery details.)

A wise father doesn't see everything.

W.A.C. BENNETT

Full Term Plus 12

If you will be giving birth in a hospital or birth center, you will need a **car seat** to transport your baby home. All states have laws requiring the use of approved infant car seats. Many new mothers are tempted to hold the baby in their arms while another person operates the car, but don't—this is very dangerous. A sudden stop might wrench your baby from your arms; a sudden impact might crush the baby between you and the dashboard. Please take no risks! Purchase and use a car seat appropriate for a newborn and wear a seat belt yourself *at all times*. **Remember that the safest place for your baby's car seat is the middle of the back seat.**

Full Term Plus 13

If you have a son, you will have to decide whether or not to have him circumcised. **Circumcision** is a religious rite carried out by the Muslim and Jewish faiths. Outside of religious tradition, circumcision has both advantages and disadvantages. The American Academy of Pediatrics indicates that the most significant advantage for newborns is a ten-fold reduction in the incidence and severity of urinary tract infections. While routine circumcision is discouraged, good foreskin hygiene is as easy to learn as brushing one's teeth. On the other hand, some people like the uniform appearance that results from circumcision even though the baby boy experiences pain during and after the procedure. **Determine what's best for you and your son.**

Full Term Plus 14

Today marks the end of the second week past due. Practitioners routinely order tests of fetal well-being for babies more than two weeks overdue. The results of those tests will help direct the course of action to follow. Sometimes labor starts spontaneously after the testing, sometimes it needs a little help, and sometimes it needs a lot of help. As always, remain calm and ask a lot of questions so you know what's going on. **It won't be long now.** ☺

Chart your waist size and weight here and on page 182.

WAIST SIZE   WEIGHT

So . . . what's your new due date?

(Enter labor and delivery details beginning on the facing page.)

The best things in life aren't things.

ANTHONY J. D'ANGELO

Labor and Delivery Details

When did your contractions become regular?

DATE

TIME OF DAY

How far apart were these first regular contractions?

Had any of these events happened yet?

CARRYING THE BABY LOW IN YOUR PELVIS?

PRESSURE OR HEAVY FEELING IN THE PELVIS?

BAG OF WATERS LEAKING OR BROKEN?

LOSS OF THE MUCUS PLUG?

FEELING OF EXTRA ENERGY?

LOSS OF WEIGHT?

QUEASINESS/NAUSEA?

Did you call your practitioner during your labor?

WHEN?

WHAT ABOUT?

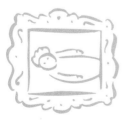

FOR BIRTH AT THE HOSPITAL

When did you leave to go to the hospital or birth center?

How did you get there?

How far apart were your contractions when you left?

What happened when you arrived?

What was it like?

FOR BIRTH AT HOME

When did your midwife arrive?

How far apart were your contractions?

What happened after the midwife arrived?

What did you do when you had contractions?

How did you manage the pain of labor?

....

....

....

....

....

....

....

....

When your contractions get to be two minutes apart,

have someone record the sequence of events and the

time at which they occur.

CLOCK TIME: EVENT:

CLOCK TIME: EVENT:

CLOCK TIME: EVENT:

CLOCK TIME: EVENT:

CLOCK TIME: EVENT:

CLOCK TIME: EVENT:

CLOCK TIME: EVENT:

CLOCK TIME: EVENT:

REFLECTIONS ON YOUR BABY'S BIRTH

Who attended the birth of your baby?

Who played the most important role?

How did the people present react to the birth?

What kinds of things happened during labor?

What was your labor like?

How long did your labor last?

Was this labor the way you imagined it would be?

How did it compare with your expectations or with

    previous labors?

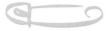

What kinds of things happened during the birth?

What was your experience of childbirth like?

Was childbirth the way you imagined it would be?

How did it compare with your expectations or with
previous births?

If you had it to do over again, what would you change
about your labor and the birth of your baby?

If you had it to do over again, what aspects of labor and
birth would you want to remain the same?

Who cut your baby's umbilical cord?

Did you hold your baby right after birth?

Describe your thoughts and reactions.

Did you try to nurse your baby right after birth?

Describe your experience.

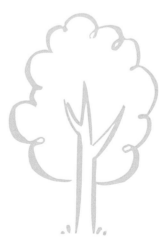

IF YOU HAD A C-SECTION

Why did you have a C-section?

_____

_____

What did the practitioner do?

_____

_____

What was the hardest part of the C-section?

_____

_____

What was the easiest part of the C-section?

_____

_____

Who was there with you during the operation?

_____

_____

Was the C-section the way you imagined it to be?

_____

_____

_____

What were the first things you noticed about your newborn baby?

_____

_____

_____

What did you do, think about, or feel right after the baby was born?

_____

_____

_____

Who were the first five people you notified with the news?

_____

_____

_____

How soon did you get up after giving birth?

_____

How long did you stay in the hospital or birth center?

_____

At home, how long did you rest before you went back to your routine?

_____

ABOUT YOUR NEW BABY

Baby's full name

How did you select your baby's name?

Date of birth

Time of birth

Weight at birth

Length at birth

What was your baby's one-minute APGAR score?

What was your baby's five-minute APGAR score?

Any hair on your baby's head? What color?

Any vernix (white, creamy material) on your baby's skin?
Where?

Any lanugo (downy hair on the body)? Where?

Any birthmarks? Where?

List any temporary changes in the baby's appearance
because of the birth (folded ear, molded head, etc.)

What did you like best about your baby's appearance?

What surprised you most about your baby's appearance?

Was your baby born before your estimated delivery date?
By how many days or weeks?

Was your baby born after your estimated delivery date?
By how many days or weeks?

What did you do the first few times you held your baby?

Breast-feeding experiences:

Bottle-feeding experiences:

Who called you "mom" for the first time? How did
you react?

What was the weather like the day your baby was born?

What local, national, or world events were in the news the day your baby was born?

Where were you living at the time?

Who were your neighbors? Your best friends?

What type of car were you driving?

What was your favorite television show?

What were your hobbies and favorite activities?

If you were employed at the time your baby was born, what was your job and who were you working for?

If you were a student at the time your baby was born, where were you going to school and how far along were you in your training?

What did you think about your whole experience of pregnancy and childbirth?

GLOSSARY & INDEX